For Elsevier:

Commissioning Editor: Mairi McCubbin
Development Editor: Sheila Black
Project Manager: Christine Johnston
Designer: Charlotte Murray, Kirsteen Wright
Illustrations Manager: Bruce Hogarth

Midwifery Essentials

Volume 3 **Labour**

Helen Baston BA(Hons) MMedSci PhD ADM PGDipEd RN RM

Lead Midwife for Education; Supervisor of Midwives, Mother & Infant Research Unit, Department of Health Sciences, University of York, York, UK

Jennifer Hall MSc ADM PGDip(HE) RN RM

Senior Lecturer in Midwifery, Faculty of Health and Life Sciences, University of the West of England, Bristol, UK

Foreword by
Jenny Fraser MSc RM RN DPSM

Lead Midwife for Risk Management and Clinical Governance, Norfolk & Norwich University Hospital NHS Foundation Trust, Norwich, UK

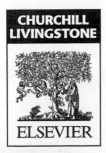

CHURCHILL LIVINGSTONE

ELSEVIER

Edinburgh London New York Oxford Philadelphia St Louis Sydney Toronto 2009

CHURCHILL
LIVINGSTONE
ELSEVIER

© 2009 Elsevier Limited. All rights reserved.

No part of this publication may be reproduced or transmitted in any form or by any means, electronic or mechanical, including photocopying, recording, or any information storage and retrieval system, without permission in writing from the publisher. Permissions may be sought directly from Elsevier's Rights Department: phone: (+1) 215 239 3804 (US) or (+44) 1865 843830 (UK); fax: (+44) 1865 853333; e-mail: healthpermissions@elsevier.com. You may also complete your request on-line via the Elsevier website at http://www.elsevier.com/permissions.

First published 2009

ISBN 978-0-443-10355-1

British Library Cataloguing in Publication Data
A catalogue record for this book is available from the British Library

Library of Congress Cataloging in Publication Data
A catalog record for this book is available from the Library of Congress

Notice
Knowledge and best practice in this field are constantly changing. As new research and experience broaden our knowledge, changes in practice, treatment and drug therapy may become necessary or appropriate. Readers are advised to check the most current information provided (i) on procedures featured or (ii) by the manufacturer of each product to be administered, to verify the recommended dose or formula, the method and duration of administration, and contraindications. It is the responsibility of the practitioner, relying on their own experience and knowledge of the patient, to make diagnoses, to determine dosages and the best treatment for each individual patient, and to take all appropriate safety precautions. To the fullest extent of the law, neither the Publisher nor the Editors assumes any liability for any injury and/or damage to persons or property arising out or related to any use of the material contained in this book.

Working together to grow
libraries in developing countries

www.elsevier.com | www.bookaid.org | www.sabre.org

ELSEVIER   BOOK AID
International   Sabre Foundation

ELSEVIER   your source for books,
journals and multimedia
in the health sciences

www.elsevierhealth.com

The
Publisher's
policy is to use
paper manufactured
from sustainable forests

Printed in Great Britain
15 14 13 12 11

Contents

All midwives strive to provide women and their families with the best-quality experience when giving birth. But what constitutes a high-quality experience? One of the perennial findings from both research and clinical experience is the value of attendant care that is attuned and sensitive. Get this right and the relationship between the mother and baby will be helped to have the best possible start. Get it wrong and there is the risk of increased distress for both. I am not saying that a woman must have a normal birth in order to achieve heightened satisfaction, although this can obviously enhance a woman's experience, but the quality of the care that she receives, whatever the type of birth, has implications for everyone's wellbeing. Responsive and sensitive communication is fundamental to good practice. If the midwife can promote and provide these conditions then the woman can be freed to draw on her own physical and personal strengths. When support is high and anxieties are reduced, she can begin labour in the right frame of mind and body.

For some time the case has been made for woman-centred care; care that is empowering, respectful and responsive. Based on the latest evidence and best clinical practice, Helen Baston and Jennifer Hall identify the key skills necessary to work with women in this way. Each page is testimony to the authors' strong beliefs that every woman deserves the highest level of care and commitment before, during and after the birth of her baby. This woman-centred philosophy applies to women whether their birth is straightforward, complicated or problematic. Their sensible, down-to-earth approach will have great appeal to all practising midwives. Student midwives are a particular target audience. If they practise as recommended, their professional careers will have the soundest of footings.

The book brings us back to basics. It is full of sense and wisdom offering a powerful reminder of the fundamental importance that our common humanity plays in this most precious of human experiences, giving birth to a new life.

Read this book eagerly, put the evidence they gather into practice without delay, and see the difference it makes.

Norwich, 2009   Jenny Fraser

To contribute to the provision of sensitive, safe and effective maternity care for women and their families is a privilege. Childbirth is a life-changing event for women. Those around them and those who input into any aspect of pregnancy, labour, birth or the postnatal period can positively influence how this event is experienced and perceived. In order to achieve this, maternity carers continually need to reflect on the services they provide and strive to keep up-to-date with developments in clinical practice. They should endeavour to ensure that women are central to the decisions made and that real choices are offered and supported by skilled practitioners.

This book is the third volume in a series of texts based on the popular 'Midwifery Basics' series published in *The Practising Midwife* journal. Since their publication, there have been many requests from students, midwives and supervisors to combine the articles into a handy text to provide a resource for learning and refreshment of midwifery knowledge and skills. The books have remained true to the original style of the articles and have been updated and expanded to create a user-friendly source of information. They are also intended to stimulate debate and require the reader both to reflect on their current practice, local policies

and procedures and to challenge care that is not woman-centred. The use of scenarios enables the practitioner to understand the context of maternity care and explore their role in its safe and effective provision.

There are many dimensions to the provision of woman-centred care that practitioners need to consider and understand. To aid this process, a jigsaw model has been introduced, with the aim of encouraging the reader to explore maternity care from a wide range of perspectives. For example, how does a midwife obtain consent from a woman for a procedure, maintain a safe environment during the delivery of care and make the most of the opportunity to promote health? What are the professional and legal issues in relation to the procedure and is this practice based on the best available evidence? Which members of the multi-professional team contribute to this aspect of care and how is it influenced by the way care is organized? Each aspect of the jigsaw should be considered during the assessment, planning, implementation and evaluation of woman-centred maternity care.

Midwifery Essentials: Labour is about the provision of safe and effective care during labour and birth. It comprises 11 chapters, each written to stand alone or be read in succession. The introductory chapter sets the scene, exploring the role of the midwife in the context of professional and national guidance. The jigsaw model for midwifery care is introduced and explained, providing a framework to explore each aspect of intrapartum care described in subsequent chapters. Chapter 2 explores assessment in early labour and the role of the midwife when a woman is admitted to the labour ward. Chapter 3 describes the first stage of labour and how the midwife monitors maternal and fetal wellbeing whilst involving the woman in decisions about her care. Chapter 4 explores how women can be enabled to cope with contractions without the use of pharmacological pain relief, and Chapter 5 builds on this, focusing specifically on the use of water to help women relax and progress throughout labour and birth. Chapter 6 focuses on the various pharmacological methods of analgesia available to women and their various advantages and disadvantages. Chapter 7 looks at the indications for induction or augmentation of labour and the impact

they might have on the woman and how she is cared for in labour. Chapter 8 discusses the role of the midwife during the second stage of labour and describes the procedure for episiotomy. Chapter 9 explores the various ways that the third stage of labour can be conducted and the impact of each method on the woman and her baby. Chapter 10 considers the indications and preparation for caesarean birth, considering the impact of different methods of anaesthesia. This volume concludes with Chapter 11, which provides a detailed account of the procedure for evidence-based perineal suturing. This book therefore prepares the reader to provide safe, evidence-based, woman-centred intrapartum care. The next book in the series explores contemporary postnatal care for women and their families, exploring the role of the midwife as a member of the multi-professional team.

	Helen Baston
York and Bristol, 2009	Jennifer Hall

Acknowledgements

In the process of writing there are always people behind the scenes who support or add to the development of the book. We would specifically like to thank Mary Seager, formerly Senior Commissioning Editor at Elsevier, for her initial vision, support and prompting to turn the journal articles from *The Practising Midwife* into a readable volume. In addition, neither of us could have completed this project without the love, support, patience and endless cups of tea and coffee provided by our partners and children. To you we owe our greatest gratitude.

Chapter 1

Introduction

This book is the third in the *Midwifery Essentials* series aimed at student midwives and those who support them in clinical practice. It focuses on intrapartum care for low-risk women beginning with how women access midwifery care; it then takes the reader through the labour journey from the onset of labour to the birth of the baby. The book concludes with a chapter on perineal repair. Scenarios are used throughout the book to facilitate learning and assist the reader to apply this knowledge to her own practice areas. The focus for contemporary maternity care is choice, access and continuity of care within a safe and effective service (Department of Health 2004, Department of Health 2007). This book explores ways in which this aspiration can become a reality for women and their families.

The aim of this introductory chapter is:

■ To introduce the 'jigsaw model' for exploring effective midwifery practice (Fig. 1.1).

The jigsaw model is used throughout the book, to examine how midwives can apply their knowledge to provide woman-centred intrapartum care.

Midwifery care model

One of the purposes of this series of books is to consider the care of women and their babies from an holistic viewpoint. This means considering the care from a physical, emotional, psychological, spiritual, social and cultural context. To do this we have developed a jigsaw model of care that will encourage the reader to consider individual aspects of midwifery care, while recognizing these aspects go to make up part of the whole person being cared for.

This model will be used to reflect on the clinical scenarios described in the chapters. It shows the dimensions of effective maternity care and each should be considered during the assessment, planning, implementation and evaluation of an aspect of care.

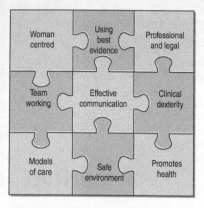

Fig. 1.1 Jigsaw model: dimensions of effective midwifery care.

The pieces of the jigsaw clearly interlink with each other and each is needed for the provision of safe, holistic intrapartum care. When one piece is missing the picture will be incomplete and care will not reach its potential. Each aspect of the model is described below in more detail. It is recommended that when an aspect of midwifery care is being evaluated, each piece of the jigsaw is addressed. Consider the questions pertaining to each piece of the jigsaw and work through those that are relevant to the clinical situation you face.

Woman-centred care

The provision of woman-centred care was one of the central messages of the policy document *Changing childbirth* (Department of Health 1993) which turned the focus of maternity care from meeting the needs of the professionals to listening and responding to the aspirations of women. This is further

enforced in the *National service framework* (Department of Health 2004) and *Maternity matters* (Department of Health 2007) and the National Institute for Health and Clinical Excellence (NICE) *Intrapartum care guidelines* (NICE 2007). The provision of woman-centred care is also an expectation of midwifery practice (NMC 2004) and pre-registration education (NMC 2009). When considering particular aspects of care the questions that need to be addressed to ensure that the woman's care is woman-centred include:

- Was the woman involved in the development of her care plan and its subsequent implementation?
- Should her family or carers also need to be involved?
- How can I ensure that she remains involved in further decisions about her care?
- What are the implications of undertaking or not undertaking this procedure on this particular woman and baby?
- Are there any factors that I need to consider that might influence the results of this procedure for this woman and their impact on her?
- How does this procedure fit in with the woman's hopes, expectations and meanings?
- Is now the most appropriate time to undertake this procedure?

Using best evidence

There is a growing body of research evidence that is available to inform the intrapartum care we provide. We have a duty to apply this knowledge, as the NMC Code states: 'you must deliver care based on the best available evidence or best practice' (NMC 2008:04). Midwifery evidence includes many aspects (Wickham 2004) and the decisions a midwife makes about her practice will be influenced by a range of factors. However, in the statement above, care should be based as much as possible on the 'best' evidence, whatever that is. Questions that need to be addressed when exploring the evidence base of care include:

- What is already known about this aspect of care?
- What is the justification for the choices made about care?
- What is the research evidence available on this procedure?
- Do local guidelines reflect best evidence?
- Was a midwife involved in development of local/national guidelines?
- Who represents users of maternity services on groups where guidelines are developed?
- What midwifery research project has your Trust been involved in?
- Where do you go first in order to identify sources of best evidence?

Professional and legal

Women need to feel confident that the midwives who care for them are working within a framework that supports safe practice. Midwives who practise in the United Kingdom must adhere to the rules and guidance of the Nursing and Midwifery Council (NMC). The Code (NMC 2008:01) states:

As a professional you are accountable for actions and omissions in your practice and must always justify your decisions. You must always act lawfully, whether those laws relate to your professional practice or personal life.

Midwives are therefore required to comply with legal statutes and the rules and regulations of their employers.

Questions that need to be addressed to ensure that the woman's care fulfils statutory obligations include:

- Is this procedure expected to be an integral part of education prior to qualification?
- How do the midwives rules relate to this care?
- Which NMC proficiencies relate to this care?
- How does the NMC Code relate to this care?
- Is there any other NMC guidance applicable to this care?
- Are there any national or international guidelines for this care?
- Are there any legal issues underpinning the use of this care?

Team working

Whilst midwives are the experts in low-risk intrapartum care, they remain reliant on a number of other workers to provide a comprehensive, safe service. Midwives work as part of a team of professional and support staff who each bring particular skills and perspectives to the care of women and their families. The NMC Code requires registrants to 'keep colleagues informed when you are sharing care with others' and 'work with colleagues to monitor the quality of your work and maintain the safety of those in your care' (2008:03). It also states:

- You must work cooperatively within teams and respect the skills, expertise and contributions of your colleagues
- You must be willing to share your skills and experience for the benefit of your colleagues
- You must consult and take advice from colleagues when appropriate
- You must treat your colleagues fairly and without discrimination (NMC 2008:03).

The midwives rules and standards also require midwives to refer any woman or baby whose condition deviates from normal to an appropriate health professional (2004:16).

Questions that need to be addressed to ensure that the woman's care makes appropriate use of the multi-professional team include:

- Does this care fall within my role?
- Have I acknowledged the limitations of my professional knowledge?
- Who else will need to be involved?
- Where should this care be recorded for all to see?
- Who will I involve if my observations are outside normal parameters?
- How can I facilitate effective team working with this woman?

- Will another person be required to assist with this care?
- When will they be available and how can I access them?

Effective communication

Providing woman-centred care to women during labour and birth requires midwives to engage and communicate effectively with them. It is essential that the midwife is aware of the cues she is giving to the woman during the care she provides. Time is often pressured in midwifery, both in the community and hospital setting, but it is important to convey to the woman that she is the focus of your attention. Taking time to explain what you are going to do, and why, is crucial if she is going to trust that you will always act in her best interest.

Questions that need to be addressed throughout intrapartum care include:

- What opportunities are there for the woman to convey her hopes and fears for the labour and birth?
- How can the midwife facilitate meaningful discussion about choices for birth?
- What information needs to be given in order for the woman to choose whether this is the right decision for her?
- How can the birth partner be effectively involved in supporting the woman?
- Has she given consent?
- Is she clear what the care entails?
- In what ways could the information be given?

- What should be said during the care?
- What should be observed in the woman's behaviour during the care?
- What should be communicated to the woman after the care?
- How and where should recording of the care and its effectiveness be made?

Clinical dexterity

Midwives providing intrapartum care need to exercise a range of skills in order to provide choice for women. They need to be able to employ competent technical knowledge when supporting a woman who requests pharmacological means of pain relief, for example, and also need to be able to adapt to provide the supportive skills needed for women who want to labour without drugs. Midwives need to apply their experience and wisdom to facilitate normal birth and have the confidence to encourage women to try alternative positions for labour and birth. The midwife continues to learn new skills throughout her working life and is accountable for maintaining and developing her practice as new ways of working are introduced (NMC 2008:04).

Questions that need to be addressed to ensure that the woman's care is provided with clinical dexterity include:

- How has practice changed since I first qualified as a midwife?
- Can I practise this skill in other ways?
- How has my previous experience influenced how I approach this procedure today?
- How can I be sure I am carrying this out correctly?

- Are there opportunities for practising this skill elsewhere?
- Who can I observe to explore alternative ways of doing this?

Models of care

One of the key policy recommendations is that women should have choice about where they give birth (Department of Health 2007). In order to facilitate this, midwives work in many settings and in a range of maternity care systems. For example, midwives work in primary care, providing home birth services and in local midwife-led units, providing home from home care for low-risk women. Midwives can also work independently providing holistic client-centred care, or within a large tertiary centre providing care for women with specific health needs. The models of care can be influential in determining the care that a woman may receive, from whom and when. Midwives need to consider the most appropriate ways that care can be delivered so that they can influence future development in the best interests of women and their families.

Questions that need to be addressed to ensure that the impact of the way that care is provided is acknowledged include:

- How long has care been provided in this way?
- How is the maternity service organized?
- Which professional groups are involved in the provision of this service?
- How is this procedure/care influenced by the model of care provided?

- How does this model of care impact on the carers?
- How does this model of care impact on the woman and her family?
- Is this the best way to provide care from a professional point of view?

Safe environment

Midwives providing intrapartum care need to ensure that the environment in which they work supports safe and effective working practices and protects the woman and her family from harm. The NMC Code states that 'you must have the skills and knowledge for safe and effective practice when working without direct supervision' (NMC 2008:04). The midwife must ensure that the care she gives does not compromise the safety of women and their families. She must therefore create and maintain a safe working environment at all times, whether in a woman's home or in a hospital service. Questions that need to be addressed to ensure that the woman's care is provided in a safe environment include:

- Can the woman be assured that her confidentiality will be maintained?
- Does the woman understand the implications of giving her consent to this procedure?
- Are there facilities to ensure that her privacy and dignity are maintained?
- Is there somewhere to wash hands?
- Is there an appropriate place to dispose of waste?
- Is the equipment appropriately maintained and free from contamination?

- Is the space adequate to allow ease of movement around the woman without invading her personal space?
- What are the risks involved in this procedure/care and how have they been addressed?
- Are there any risks to the person undertaking this procedure/care?
- Is this environment safe for others who might come into the room?

Promotes health

Providing intrapartum care for women and their families presents a unique opportunity to influence the health and wellbeing of the public. Midwives must capitalize on their contacts with women to help them achieve a safe and fulfilling labour and birth and promote lifestyle choices that will benefit women, babies and families in the future. Questions that need to be addressed to ensure that the woman's care promotes health include:

- Is this procedure/care going to help her or harm her or her baby in any way?
- What are the opportunities to use this procedure to educate her/her family on healthy behaviours?
- What resources can women and families access to help them make healthy lifestyle choices?
- Has enough time been allocated to this aspect of care to make the most of the opportunities to promote healthy living?
- Who else should I involve to ensure that the woman and her family get the best possible advice in this situation?

The book begins with a chapter focusing on how women access maternity care, using the jigsaw model to examine how the midwife can provide holistic care. The subsequent chapters also use the jigsaw model to explore scenarios from practice, focusing on the role of the midwife in the various aspects of intrapartum care. Thus the reader is provided with a structure with which to reflect on her care and that of the multi-professional team in which she works. Each chapter includes a range of activities designed to enable the midwife to contextualize the information within her own practice, applying her continually developing knowledge to her own circumstances. The chapters are written so that they can be accessed without having read the previous ones, although we hope you will find the whole book relevant and thought provoking. Enjoy!

References

Department of Health: *Changing childbirth: report of the expert maternity group pt. II, Report of the Expert Maternity Group Pt.1*. London, 1993, Department of Health.

Department of Health: *National service framework for children, young people and maternity services*. Standard 11. 2004, Maternity Services.

Department of Health: *Maternity matters: choice, access and continuity of care in a safe service*, London, 2007, Department of Health.

National Institute for Health and Clinical Excellence (NICE): *Intrapartum care. Care of healthy women and their babies during childbirth. NICE clinical guideline 55*, London, 2007, NICE.

Nursing and Midwifery Council (NMC): *Midwives rules and standards*, London, 2004, NMC.

Nursing and Midwifery Council (NMC): *The code. Standards of conduct, performance and ethics for nurses and midwives*, London, 2008, NMC.

Nursing and Midwifery Council (NMC): *Standards for pre-registration midwifery education*, London, 2009, NMC.

Wickham S: Feminism and ways of knowing. In Stewart M, editor: *Pregnancy, birth and maternity care: feminist perspectives*, Oxford, 2004, Books for Midwives, pp 157–168.

Chapter 2

Early assessment and admission in labour

Trigger scenario

Clare is at home experiencing painful uterine contractions. She is 39 weeks pregnant and expecting her first baby. She is unsure about when she should come into hospital – her partner is worried about the traffic and does not want to leave it too late.

Introduction

The early stages of labour may be a challenging time for many women, especially with their first baby. Fear and anxiety will play a part in the woman's ability to cope, especially if she is alone and unsure what is happening. If she is having community-based care she will have an on-call system where she may contact a midwife for help and advice. If she is planning a hospital birth she will be given a telephone number for the labour ward to contact for advice. In some hospitals this is a special area where assessment may take place (Morgan 2007). These calls should normally be answered by a qualified midwife though students should have opportunity in their education programme to gain experience in speaking to labouring women on the phone. This chapter is more focused on the hospital situation, though the principles also apply for assessment in the home situation.

Activity

Consider where assessment of labour takes place in your area.
Find out who usually answers the telephone.
Find out how the conversation is documented.

The stage at which a woman goes into hospital could have a significant impact on her labour experience (Rahnama & Faghigzadeh 2006). If she goes in too early, at a time when she is in pain and vulnerable, she may ask for or accept analgesia sooner than she otherwise might. Also, the longer she is on the hospital birth suite, the less likely she is to experience continuity of carer. However, many women lack confidence to stay at home and want to have access to midwifery care 'just in case' (Cheyne et al 2007).

The midwife who answers the telephone has a complex role to fulfil. She must rule out conditions that make admission to hospital advisable and, at the same time, instil confidence in the woman to stay at home longer if labour is not yet established. The response that the woman receives when she telephones the hospital birth suite is important for many reasons. She is potentially speaking to the midwife who will care for her when she is admitted, and the impression she forms following this interaction has the potential to relieve or raise anxiety.

For many women, hospital is seen as a place of safety when labour begins (Cheyne et al 2007). The hospital birth suite is the place where she has often imagined herself during her mental preparation for the birth of her baby. To gain admission is to acknowledge that labour has really begun and that the unknown becomes a reality.

Home assessment

Women in early labour should have access to midwifery support and advice (Baxter 2007). In ideal circumstances, this care is provided in the woman's own home by her community midwife, enabling her to remain in familiar surroundings for longer (Flint 1984). In some areas women do not decide where they will labour and birth until it begins and the midwife assesses them at home (Leap & Edwards 2006:110). However, access to such a service is limited and may not be available to all groups of women, for example high-risk women or those with complex social needs.

In a multi-centre trial conducted in Canada (Janssen et al 2006) comparing home assessment with telephone triage, women who were assessed at home were less likely to be admitted to the labour ward with cervical dilatation of 3 cm or less, but there was no impact on the caesarean section rates. Recent randomised controlled trials of structured support in early labour suggest that women value and are highly satisfied with this service, but that there is little impact on clinical outcomes (Spiby & Renfrew 2008).

Further research is required in this area to look at specific and targeted support for particular groups of women who may benefit from additional care during early labour.

Communication by telephone

Face-to-face communication is the most effective means of sending and receiving messages. Our body language transmits so much more than our spoken words. When communicating by telephone, this aspect is not available and the midwife must pay particular attention to the tone, rate and timing of the spoken word, as well as the content of the conversation. This paralanguage has been described as 'the vocal cues which accompany spoken words' (Rungapadiachy 1999:210).

It is important that the midwife talks with the woman and not her partner or friend, as this can lead to a three-way conversation. There is then the potential for the middle person to either misinterpret the question the midwife asks or to reword what the woman says, leading to an inaccurate portrayal of events. Also, when the midwife speaks directly with the woman, she is able to assess how she is coping by her tone of voice. However, if a woman is in severe pain, or in water, she may be unable to reach a phone easily and her partner should not be ignored as some women may have rapid labours and births. Box 2.1 summarizes the 10 steps to be taken when talking to labouring women on the telephone.

Step 1: Confirm name and hospital number

The conversation should begin with the midwife introducing herself, and then confirming the woman's name and hospital number. Asking for her number near the beginning of the conversation will also prompt the woman to bring her maternity records to the telephone. Confirmation of her name and number will also enable the midwife to access the correct woman's hospital records in preparation for her admission.

Step 2: Confirm address

The woman's location is required. It is essential that the correct address is written down and repeated back to her, especially in the event that she requires transport into hospital via ambulance. Her details will be given to an ambulance control operator and then to the ambulance crew. There is a possibility that information can be misheard; hence, it is important to start with the correct details to avoid delay.

Step 3: Confirm gestation and parity

If the woman is experiencing painful contractions before full term, she will need to be admitted without delay. There may be the possibility that labour can be delayed with the use of tocolytic therapy, depending on gestation and estimated fetal weight, although this course of action needs to be weighed carefully against the side-effects of the drugs used (Jordan 2002).

A woman who has already experienced a vaginal birth is likely to progress more quickly in labour than a primigravida, and this should be considered when giving advice, though this is not always the case.

Step 4: Assess recent pregnancy history

The woman should be asked about her general health and wellbeing during her pregnancy. Has she had any infections or worries about the baby's growth or movements? She will be able to say from her maternity records (if she is unable to remember) what the presentation is and what her blood pressure has been. If she has had a previous caesarean section, she will also require close monitoring

Box 2.1 Ten steps for giving telephone advice to a labouring woman

1. **Confirm name and hospital number**
Rationale For identification purposes and also to enable the woman to be addressed by name during the conversation. If admission is recommended, it is also important that she is greeted by name on arrival

2. **Confirm address**
Rationale For identification purposes. Also necessary if an ambulance is required and to be aware of the distance to be travelled

3. **Confirm gestation and parity**
Rationale Essential information required to contextualize subsequent information

4. **Assess recent pregnancy history**
Rationale Need to identify if there is a reason why admission should not be delayed

5. **Assess recent medical history**
Rationale Need to identify if there is a reason why admission should not be delayed

6. **Obtain history or reason for call**
Rationale Identify nature of presenting concern(s)

7. **Assess which coping strategies have been tried**
Rationale To identify what other strategies to suggest

8. **Outline the options available**
Rationale To empower the woman to make a decision that reflects her current needs

9a. **If the woman decides to stay at home, inform her of when she should ring again**
Rationale To provide clear criteria of when admission is recommended and to enable her to feel comfortable to ring again at any time if she needs further advice

9b. **If the woman decides to come in, confirm transport arrangements and remind her to bring her maternity records**
Rationale To establish if an ambulance is required. To ensure that the woman brings her maternity records

10. **Document advice given as per hospital policy**
Rationale To provide record of advice given to inform future conversations. To provide useful audit information to inform future maternity services

during labour, although the rate of uterine rupture is 0.3 per cent, according to a multi-centre study (Appleton et al 2000).

Step 5: Assess recent medical history

It is important to know if the woman has any underlying medical condition that will require close monitoring during labour, such as diabetes, hypertension or infection.

Step 6: Obtain history or reason for call

There will be a particular event or combination of events that has caused the woman to seek advice from the midwife or hospital delivery suite. In relation to diagnosis of labour, the midwife will need to assess when contractions started, how long they last and how frequently they are occurring.

The key to assessing that labour is progressing is that contractions are becoming more frequent, progressively more painful and lasting longer. If the woman thinks that her membranes may have ruptured, she is advised to come into hospital for confirmation. At term, in the absence of meconium-stained liquor, contractions or evidence of infection, some maternity units send women back home to await events. However, it has been suggested (Hannah et al 2000) that expectant management at home increases the risk of some adverse outcomes following the rupturing of membranes and women should be advised:

- 'The risk of serious neonatal infection is 1% rather than 0.5% for women with intact membranes
- 60% of women with prelabour rupture of the membranes will go into labour within 24 hours

- Induction of labour is appropriate approximately 24 hours after rupture of the membranes.' (NICE 2007: 22–23)

Step 7: Assess which coping strategies have been tried

There are many different scenarios for the use of coping strategies. The woman may have attended preparation for childbirth classes and considered the use of non-pharmacological means to alleviate pain in labour. Thus, she might ring the hospital birth suite having tried and used them all, with good effect, and hence be in established labour.

Alternatively, she may have tried some and found little benefit. She may feel she needs additional support. On the other hand, a woman might not know how to cope with contractions at home and may benefit from some simple advice. Thus, the midwife must assess what the woman has tried before she gives further advice.

Step 8: Outline the options available

The midwife needs to assimilate all the information she has gleaned from the conversation and assess the need for admission. She will then present the alternatives back to the woman in a balanced way. The woman should be in no doubt about what is recommended – for example, admission if spontaneous rupture of membranes is suspected. However, if it appears that birth is not imminent, and there are no medical or obstetric risk factors, she has the option of staying at home longer if she wishes.

Step 9a: If the woman decides to stay at home, inform her of when she should ring again

Unless there is a situation requiring urgent attention, such as evidence of second stage of labour or bleeding, a woman who feels confident to stay at home until labour becomes more established should be reassured that she can ring back for further advice at any time. She must be advised to ring back if she experiences any fresh vaginal bleeding, spontaneous rupture of membranes, constant abdominal pain or the need for analgesia.

Step 9b: If a woman decides to come in, confirm transport arrangements and remind her to bring her maternity records

Unless there is an emergency situation, such as indication of second stage, bleeding or prematurity, there is usually no reason why the woman cannot make her own way to hospital in private transport. If she does not have a car, a neighbour or friend might be delighted to be chosen to stand by to take her to the hospital birth suite.

Women can be advised antenatally that a trial run is a useful exercise, bearing in mind traffic at peak times and where the nearest hospital car park is. The labouring woman should not drive herself to hospital.

Step 10: Document advice given as per hospital policy

It is practice in some maternity units to document all telephone advice.

This can provide valuable information in the event of a woman ringing again after a change of shift. If the midwife who took the initial call is still on duty then, where possible, it would be advantageous for both woman and midwife if the continuity of care was maintained.

The same midwife will be able to detect from the woman's voice if there has been a change either in her progress in labour or her level of anxiety. The records will prompt the midwife to ask questions that build on previous interaction, confirming to the woman that she is being cared for as an individual. For example, 'Did you have a bath? Did it help your backache?' Such records have the potential to be a valuable data-collection tool for use in clinical audit. A study looking at the use of the telephone advice documentation used in the All Wales clinical pathway for normal labour (Spiby et al 2006) showed that women were satisfied with this service if they had been given a choice about coming into hospital and were made welcome to do so; if they were told when they should phone back and if they were treated in a friendly and encouraging manner. They were likely to feel dissatisfied, however, if the midwife whom they had spoken to previously had not passed on information, if they did not feel treated with respect, if their worries were not alleviated by the phone call or if they did not receive clear guidance.

Admission to the hospital birth suite

In ideal circumstances, when the woman has decided to come into hospital, a midwife will be allocated to her care. This midwife will ensure that a room is prepared for her admission and that, when the woman arrives, she and others know where her room is. It is likely that the woman will feel anxious on admission; she will be anticipating an uncertain future. If she is greeted with a smile and a personal welcome, she is more likely to feel valued and respected.

The midwife must assess the woman's condition as soon as possible. Is birth imminent and/or does she have any vaginal loss? If the woman is not pushing with contractions and any vaginal loss is clear, further assessment can continue at a more leisurely pace.

Ideally, subsequent assessment should consist of exploring her story and her antenatal records with her and observing how she responds to any contractions. This observation is ongoing during the important baseline observations of temperature, pulse and blood pressure. The midwife will assess what has brought the woman to seek admission to the hospital. She will build up a picture of when contractions started, when they became regular, and if there has been any vaginal loss. A specimen of urine should be requested and routine urinalysis performed. The midwife should acknowledge the woman's birth plan and continue the discussion as labour progresses.

Women should be encouraged to wear their own clothes during their hospital stay, to have their belongings around them and use their own toiletries. Nightclothes suggest inactivity and peaceful slumber, rather than the activity and hard work that comes with childbirth. A large cotton T-shirt, worn with tracksuit bottoms or shorts, would perhaps be more suitable attire for activity. The bottom half can be discarded as labour progresses.

Observation of mood continues during abdominal palpation to confirm gestational age, lie, presentation and degree of engagement. The fetal heart should be auscultated for a full minute after a contraction and, if possible, during one, and the maternal pulse assessed at the same time (NICE 2007:144).

The midwife should also have the skill of detecting uterine contractions abdominally, without the use of an abdominal transducer. By gently placing a calm hand on the uterine fundus the midwife can chat with the woman and assess uterine and fetal activity at the same time. When a contraction begins, the midwife should stop talking and check both the time (e.g. 15:13 hours) and observe the length of the contraction in seconds. Assessing the strength of the contraction abdominally is an imprecise science. Fortunately, the woman can usually provide this information herself, unless she has had an epidural or narcotic. To assess the frequency of contractions, the midwife should stay with the woman for at least three contractions.

Vaginal examination

Unless there is an absolute indication (to confirm an uncertain presentation) and the fetal heart is within normal parameters, then vaginal examination may be delayed until the woman has become more acclimatized to her new surroundings. If no action is to be taken on the findings, the examintion is unnecessary. However, progress in labour is often described by the dilatation (in centimetres) of the cervical os and the woman may want and expect this information soon after admission.

The steps in the procedure for vaginal examination are outlined in Box 2.2. Though this describes a particular method of hygiene steps, the midwife should check what is expected in the policies of her local unit including the types of gloves to be used. Mary Stewart (2005) highlights that this method of hygiene could be regarded as an issue of power and control and that women could be enabled to clean themselves if required. NICE intrapartum care guidelines (2007) recognize the need for more research around hygiene care behaviours in labour. It is particularly important, as outlined by Crompton (1996), that permission is sought before examination and that the woman is reassured that it will stop whenever she wishes. If a contraction occurs during the examination, the midwife should pause and assess how the presenting part applies to the cervix, but keep her fingers still. The fingers should not be removed until the procedure is complete to avoid introducing infection.

Once the examination is over, the fetal heart must then be re-auscultated. The woman is made comfortable, with the option to get dressed again if appropriate. The woman needs feedback about what the examination found and what the implications are for her immediate care (Olsen 2006). The use of appropriate language to describe what has been found is essential (Stewart 2005). Documenting the findings by her bedside provides an ideal opportunity for this.

With woman

Although the ideal scenario of continuity of one-to-one care is that which is both presented here and recommended by the Department of

Box 2.2 Procedure for vaginal examination

- Explain the nature of the procedure and why it is required

Rationale So that the woman knows what to expect and understands what information the procedure will provide

- Obtain verbal consent

Rationale To ensure that the procedure is undertaken with the woman's agreement

- Ask the woman to empty her bladder

Rationale To avoid discomfort during the procedure and to avoid distortion of fundal height

- Undertake abdominal palpation (for procedure, see Baston & Hall 2009)

Rationale To provide additional confirmation for VE findings. To ensure normal fetal heart rate prior to procedure

- Provide opportunity for birth partner to leave or stay

Rationale To avoid embarrassment for either woman or birth partner

- Ask woman to remove pants while equipment is gathered, providing modesty sheet

Rationale To maintain privacy and dignity

- Gather VE pack (sterile sheets, hand towel, gallipot, sanitary towel, cotton wool swabs), sterile gloves, lubricant cream/jelly and tissues

Rationale To avoid leaving the woman to seek additional equipment during the procedure

- Wash and dry hands

Rationale To avoid cross-infection

- Open pack, fold back paper to create clean field, place bag nearby to use for disposal of swabs, open gloves onto clean field, squirt lubricant into gallipot (a small plastic receiver), fill other pot with tap water to prepare equipment prior to donning sterile gloves

Rationale To prepare for the procedure and avoid having to break off to find equipment

- Ensure woman is comfortable in semi-recumbent position on bed or mattress, with slight left lateral tilt

Rationale To avoid vena-caval compression due to weight of gravid uterus

- Wash hands and dry with sterile towel from pack, don gloves

Rationale To avoid cross-infection

- Ask woman to draw up knees and let legs flop outward to allow vulval area to be swabbed. Place sterile waterproof sheet under woman's bottom and second one on her abdomen

Rationale To avoid soiling the bed, and to provide a local sterile field

- Swabbing: If right-handed, use right hand to soak swab with tap water and transfer to left hand to swab outer aspect of left labia majora, from top down in one movement. Discard swab in bag. Repeat swabbing: right labia majora, left then right labia minora, and finally introitus

Rationale To avoid contamination of clean area. Observation of the genitalia (scarring, varicosities or oedema) also takes place during swabbing

continued

Box 2.2 Continued

• Wait until after a contraction, dip index and middle fingers of right hand (if right-handed) in lubricating cream, gently part labia with thumb and finger of left hand and gently introduce lubricated fingers in downward and backward direction

Rationale To avoid unneccessary discomfort. To follow natural curve of vagina to avoid discomfort

• Gentle digital examination of cervix and presenting part, giving feedback to the woman as appropriate

Rationale To estimate the effacement and dilatation of the cervix, the position of the fetus and station of the presenting part (Figs 2.1 and 2.2)

• Remove fingers, dry vulval region and position new sanitary towel. Remove gloves, ensure modesty sheet is in position and auscultate the fetal heart. Clear away equipment

Rationale To make woman comfortable and ensure fetal wellbeing

• Document the examination, noting date and time; indication; health of external genitalia; effacement, dilatation and application of cervix; presence of forewaters; station, identity, moulding and position of presenting part; vaginal loss; and fetal heart rate. Add signature

Rationale To provide a record of the rationale for the examination and its findings

---

Health (2007), in reality, midwives often care for more than one woman in labour. Although a midwife may have been allocated a woman in active labour and one in early labour, the situation can change at any point during labour, with the potential for both to require a lot of support simultaneously. Inevitably, there will be times when the midwife needs to leave the room. The woman and her partner should be shown how to summon help if they require it and that they must do so even if the midwife has only briefly left the room.

It is vital that the midwife keeps the coordinating midwife informed of the progress of the women in her care. Any change in condition, concern or uncertainty should be reported to the

senior midwife and recorded as soon as possible.

Activity

Revise the indications for vaginal examination during labour.
   Think about when vaginal examination by a midwife is contraindicated.

Admission cardiotocography

The use of electronic fetal monitoring (EFM) to provide an admission trace has been part of routine midwifery practice in many maternity units in the UK. However, this practice has not been advocated for low-risk women since 2001 (NICE 2001) and subsequent

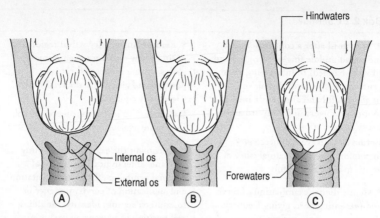

Fig. 2.1 Effacement of the cervix. (Adapted from Johnson & Taylor 2006, with permission.)

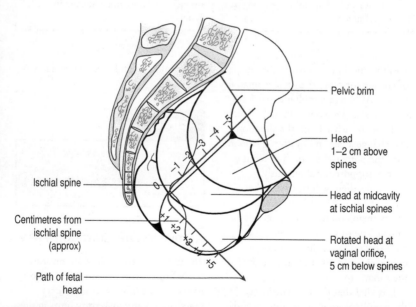

Fig. 2.2 Level of presenting part in relation to the ischial spines. (Adapted from Johnson & Taylor 2006, with permission.)

guidance has maintained this stance (NICE 2007:170):

The use of admission cardiotocography (CTG) in low-risk pregnancy is not recommended in any birth setting.

The woman should be involved in the decision about how her baby is monitored. She should have had access to the information she needs to make an informed choice during the antenatal period. However, the amount or nature of the information may be overwhelming for her, and she may need to clarify issues with the midwife before she makes her choice. Although the evidence does not support the use of routine continuous EFM for low-risk women, the situation can change during the labour.

Activity

Find out what the NICE guidelines (2007) recommend for fetal heart rate monitoring during the first stage of labour.

Consider the circumstances which would lead the midwife to recommend to the woman that the fetus should be monitored continuously.

Reflection on trigger scenario

Look back on the trigger scenario at the start of the chapter.

Clare is at home experiencing painful uterine contractions. She is 39 weeks pregnant and expecting her first baby. She is unsure about when she should come into hospital – her partner is worried about the traffic and does not want to leave it too late.

Now that you are familiar with care in the early stages of labour you should have insight into how the scenario relates to the evidence. The jigsaw model will now be used to explore the trigger scenario in more depth.

Effective communication

Responding to telephone calls from women in early labour is a common activity on busy labour wards. In this situation Clare is unsure about what to do and it is probable that she will telephone for advice. Questions that arise include: Where will she call and who will answer the telephone? What questions will be asked in order for the midwife to assess if she needs to go to hospital yet? How will she be reassured? What information will be provided so that she can make the right choice appropriate to her? How can the midwife be sure she is giving the correct information?

Woman-centred care

In early labour midwives need to ensure women are enabled to make the most appropriate decision for them. Their anxieties and fears should be addressed and they should be empowered in their choices. Questions that may be asked include: Has Clare created a birth plan for labour with her midwife? What plans has she made for labour? Is an invitation to attend the birth unit appropriate at this time for Clare and her partner? If she does not come in now what advice will be given about when to attend? How do the suggestions made about staying at home or coming into the unit fit in with Clare's hopes, expectations and meanings?

Using best evidence

In this situation evidence surrounding communication and procedures in early labour will be helpful. Local evidence about distance from the unit and traffic may also influence the information given and the choices made. Questions that could be asked include: What is the evidence around length of first stage of labour for women experiencing a first labour? What information will be required from Clare to establish how far in labour she may be? What does the evidence say about the disadvantages of coming into hospital before labour is established? What are the local guidelines and on what evidence are these based?

Professional and legal

Midwives need to be aware of their roles and responsibilities in early labour related to the rules and codes of practice (NMC 2004, 2008). A midwife's behaviour and attitude is just as important as if she is face to face. Questions that are relevant include: Has the midwife received training around communication on the telephone in early labour through her initial education programme prior to qualification? Has she received any ongoing training as updating? How does this situation relate to the rule of practice? How does the code of ethics

and professional conduct relate to this situation? Are there any national or international guidelines for this procedure? Are there any legal issues relating to this situation?

Team working

In this scenario the midwife will need to work as a team with Clare and her partner in order to make the appropriate choices for Clare. There may be other members of the team that the midwife will need to inform of Clare's impending arrival in the unit. Questions that could be asked include: Who should be answering the telephone? Who else may need to be involved in Clare's care? Where should the conversation be recorded? Who will be involved should Clare's history be complicated? Who will care for Clare when she arrives on the labour ward?

Clinical dexterity

When assessing a woman in early labour the midwife uses a range of clinical skills. She will need to take an accurate history and be able to perform abdominal palpation, fetal heart rate auscultation and vaginal examination as well as base line observations. Questions that may arise include: How will the midwife's previous experience influence how she approaches Clare and her need for information? How often is the midwife rostered to provide intrapartum care? How does she maintain and develop her clinical skills? What should she do if she performs an examination but is unsure of her findings?

Models of care

In this scenario Clare is intending to go into hospital to receive care. In this model of care Clare will be unlikely to have met the midwife she is going to speak to on the telephone. Questions that may arise include: Are there any challenges for Clare in the way that the services are organized? How does this model of care impact on the midwife? How does this model of care impact on Clare's partner? How can maternity services be organized to facilitate continuity of care? Does Clare's community midwife undertake intrapartum care?

Safe environment

Clare is in her own environment but to receive care in this situation she will need to transfer to the hospital. Safety will involve her being supported to make the right choice to attend the hospital not too early but also not so far in labour that she and her partner are very stressed or anxious. Questions that could arise include: Is confidentiality maintained throughout the discussion on the telephone? What are the risks involved to Clare, her baby and partner through making the choice to stay at home or to drive to the hospital?

Promotes health

In considering whether to advise Clare to stay at home or to come into hospital the midwife should be assessing the effect on Clare's wellbeing. Questions that may arise include: Can the midwife promote her self-esteem

and wellbeing by supporting Clare to stay home for longer? Will staying at home be more stressful than coming into the hospital? Will this in the long term be more harmful to Clare and her baby?

Further scenarios

The following scenarios enable you to consider how specific situations influence the care the midwife provides. Use the jigsaw model to explore the issues raised in each scenario.

Scenario 1

Valerie has been called to Jamelia's home, where she has started having regular contractions in the past hour. This is her first baby and she is planning to use a pool for a home birth. When she arrives Jamelia is in pain and asks if she can get in the water.

Practice point

Caring for women in labour is not an exact science and women do not always conform to expected parameters. Therefore individual needs should be met. In this situation it is not clear how far the labour has progressed, but consideration should be given to Jamelia's needs and choices, as well as evidence around care in labour.

Further questions specific to Scenario 1 include:

1. What questions should Valerie ask Jamelia about her current feelings and experience?

2. What observations should she make to assess what is happening?

3. Where should the information be documented?

4. What are the usual parameters of time for a woman experiencing her first labour?

5. What is the evidence around the use of water in labour?

6. Can Valerie support Jamelia in other ways prior to getting in the pool?

7. Does it matter if she gets in the pool now, if it makes her comfortable?

8. Where will Valerie document the information she has obtained?

Scenario 2

Tina has arrived at the labour unit. It is her third baby and she had a caesarean section for her first birth. She has been having contractions regularly for about 5 hours and they are now about 3 minutes apart. She is breathing through the contractions but she has had a bright red vaginal blood loss that is soaking onto her pad.

Practice point

In situations where women are experiencing blood loss midwives need to ensure appropriate assessment takes place. In Tina's situation it is not clear whether she is in the latter stages of

labour or where the bleeding is coming from.

Further questions specific to Scenario 2 include:

1. What could the blood loss signal?

2. What questions will the midwife need to ask Tina?

3. What immediate observations will she make to establish the wellbeing of Tina and her baby?

4. Who will the midwife need to inform of her findings if they are unusual?

5. How will the midwife communicate what is happening to Tina?

6. Should she carry out a vaginal examination?

Conclusion

Admission to the hospital delivery suite of a woman in labour is a significant part of the labour continuum. To her, it marks the imminent arrival of the baby. The admitting midwife can make a significant impact on the woman's confidence and ability to make important decisions about her care, and can help her cope with painful uterine contractions. The midwife must develop and employ a range of technical and interpersonal skills in order to maximize the woman's experience.

Useful resources

Association of Radical Midwives: Invaders of privacy. http://www.radmid. demon.co.uk/Privacy.htm.

Baby centre: http://www.babycentre. co.uk/pregnancy/labourandbirth/ labour/admissionprocedures/.

Emma's diary: http://www.emmasdiary. co.uk/pregnancy//article/other_useful_ pregnancy_info/article/Labour_and_ birth.

References

Appleton B, Targett C, Rasmussen M, et al: Vaginal birth after caesarean section: an Australian multicentre study, BAC Study Group, *Australian and New Zealand Journal of Obstetrics and Gynaecology* 40(1):87–91, 2000.

Baston H, Hall J: *Midwifery essentials: antenatal*, Edinburgh, 2009, Elsevier.

Baxter J: Care during the latent phase of labour: supporting normal birth, *British Journal of Midwifery* 15(12):765–767, 2007.

Cheyne H, Terry R, Niven C, et al: 'Should I come in now?': a study of women's early labour experiences, *British Journal of Midwifery* 15(10):604–609, 2007.

Crompton J: Post-traumatic stress disorder and childbirth, *British Journal of Midwifery* 4(6):290–293, 1996.

Department of Health: *Maternity matters: choice, access and continuity of care in a safe service*, London, 2007, Department of Health.

Flint C: *Sensitive midwifery*, Oxford, 1984, Butterworth Heinemann.

Hannah ME, Hodnett ED, Foster WA, et al: Prelabour rupture of the membranes at term: expectant management at home or hospital? The Term PROM Study Group, *Obstetrics & Gynecology* 96(4):533–538, 2000.

Janssen P, Still D, Klein M, et al: Early labour care at home versus telephone triage, *Obstetrics & Gynecology* 108(6):1463–1469, 2006.

Johnson R, Taylor W: *Skills for midwifery practice*, ed 2, Edinburgh, 2006, Elsevier.

Jordan S: *Pharmacology for midwives: the evidence base for safe practice*, Basingstoke, 2002, Palgrave.

Leap N, Edwards N: The politics of involving women in decision making. In Page L, McCandlish R, editors: *The new midwifery: science and sensitivity in practice*, ed 2, Edinburgh, 2006, Chruchill Livingstone.

Morgan J: Delivery suite assessment unit: auditing innovation in maternity triage, *British Journal of Midwifery* 15(8):506–510, 2007.

National Institute for Health and Clinical Excellence (NICE): *The use of electronic fetal monitoring. The use and interpretation of cardiotocography in intrapartum fetal surveillance. Inherited Clinical Guideline C*, London, 2001, NICE.

National Institute for Health and Clinical Excellence (NICE): *Intrapartum care of healthy women and their babies during childbirth. NICE Clinical Guideline 55*, London, 2007, NICE.

Nursing and Midwifery Council (NMC): *Midwives rules and standards*, London, 2004, NMC.

Nursing and Midwifery Council (NMC): *The Code. Standards of conduct, performance and ethics for nurse and midwives*, London, 2008, NMC.

Olsen K: Vaginal examination: learning from experience, *The Practising Midwife* 9(6):24–25, 2006.

Rahnama P, Ziaei S, Faghigzadeh S: Impact of early admission in labour on method of delivery, *International Journal of Obstetrics and Gynecology* 92(3): 217–220, 2006.

Rungapadiachy D: *Interpersonal communication and psychology for healthcare professionals*, Oxford, 1999, Butterworth Heinemann.

Spiby H, Green JM, Hucknall C, et al: Labouring to better effect: studies of services for women in early labour. The OPAL Study. Final report to the NHS service delivery and organisation of care programme (SDO/64/2003). Mother and Infant Research Unit, University of York, 2006, Dept of Health Sciences.

Spiby H, Renfrew M: Achieving the best from care in early labour, *British Medical Journal* 337:618, 2008. Editorial. Online. Available http://www.bmj.com/cgi/section_pdf/337/aug28_1/a1165.pdf. December 5.

Stewart M: 'I'm just going to wash you down': sanitizing the vaginal examination, *Journal of Advanced Nursing* 51(6):587–594, 2005.

Chapter 3

The first stage of labour

Trigger scenario

Chloe had been experiencing painful uterine contractions for 10 hours with her first baby. She had been in hospital for 6 hours, and the midwife who had been caring for her was now going off duty. The midwife had handed over Chloe's care to a midwife who would also be looking after another woman in early labour. The midwife entered the room and said, 'Hello, I'm Margaret, I'm just going to put you on the monitor.'

Introduction

Care of a woman in labour must be carefully tailored to take her individuality into account. Although labour has been neatly packaged and presented to maternity care professionals as usually taking a particular course, the specific elements that might influence that course are unique to each woman. Such factors might include the position,

gestation and presentation of the fetus as well as the parity, age and height of the woman. There are many other physical characteristics that could potentially influence the progress of the labour, and these can combine in a multitude of ways.

The midwife must also acknowledge the unique personality and history of the woman to understand how she might be feeling in order to provide care that is appropriate and sensitive. This chapter encourages the student midwife to provide woman-focused, knowledgeable care and builds on from Chapter 2. The management of labour pain is addressed in Chapters 4, 5 and 6.

Home from home

Women should be encouraged to stay at home during early labour. Newburn (2003) describes aspects of the birth environment that women find helpful during the birth. These include: space to move around, nearby toilet and bath, comfortable bed, low/adjustable lighting, and privacy and quiet. The best place in which these elements can be achieved are in the woman's home or in a midwife-led unit, if she has access to one.

A systematic review of the settings for birth concluded that there may be some benefits from home-like birth settings, including reduced likelihood of intervention and increased satisfaction (Hodnett et al 2004). Conventional labour wards are often designed with the professionals rather than the women who use them in mind. Women may not feel that they have much control over who enters the room or how it is arranged.

Admission to hospital also brings with it the expectation that the birth is imminent, yet this may not be the case. Women need to have the knowledge that the latent phase of labour can be prolonged, and that it is not a time for clock-watching. Birth partners also need this information. During a visit to the Netherlands, a midwifery colleague told me that some men were becoming so obsessed with noting the time of every contraction that one had even recorded uterine activity on a computer spreadsheet!

Listening to women

Not all maternity units place great emphasis on the use of birth plans during labour, although some do encourage them and see them as an effective means of discussing the various options that a woman might face during her labour. Whichever approach is employed in the unit where you work, it is important to ask the woman if she has completed a birth plan, as she may have spent a lot of thought and time writing down her expectations for the labour. Reading it and discussing it with her will give her confidence that she will be treated as an individual, and that you are aware of her hopes and concerns.

Women differ in the degree of control they want, but it is an increasing expectation (Green & Baston 2004). Weaver (1998) suggests that to describe women as wanting high or low levels of control is simplistic because they may have strong views about one aspect of their labour and lukewarm views about others. The woman should be assured that she will be consulted about all aspects of her labour care, but this must not be an empty promise.

The midwife can help the woman to feel in control and active during her labour. This activity should not be confined to physically moving about and changing position, but should extend to an active involvement in controlling her environment and care. Feeling in control during labour is significantly related to psychological wellbeing postnatally (Green et al 1998, Green & Baston 2003).

Activity

Consult Hodnett et al (2007). 'Continuous support for women during childbirth.' Cochrane Review. Identify the benefits of continuous support during labour.

Support during labour

One-to-one midwifery support to women in active labour is widely advocated (Department of Health 2007a, Department of Health 2007b, Maternity Care Working Party 2007, NICE 2007, King's Fund 2008, Royal College of Obstetricians & Gynaecologists 2008). Continuous support for women during labour, particularly by women not employed by the hospital, has been associated with increased likelihood of shorter labours and spontaneous birth, use of less

analgesia, increased satisfaction (Hodnett et al 2007). Almost all women (94%) are accompanied by a friend or relative during labour (Redshaw et al 2007). In a national survey of women's experiences of maternity care (Commission for Healthcare Audit & Inspection 2007:08) 15% of women said that they and their partner had been left alone in labour at a time when it worried them. Midwives therefore need to facilitate continuous support wherever possible, in order to improve birth outcomes for women and their babies.

The midwife

In a phenomenological study exploring the woman's encounter with the midwife during childbirth, Berg et al (1996) concluded that the presence of the midwife was the central theme. This 'presence' encompassed the need to be seen as an individual, to have a trusting relationship and to be supported and guided. Although the word midwife means 'with woman', women are able to perceive the difference between a midwife who is in the room but focusing on other tasks rather than on her, and the midwife who is there for her. Osterman & Schwartz-Barcott (1996) described 'presence' as a measure of the focus of the carer's energy and the quality and nature of the interaction. Not perceiving the midwife as supportive is a significant factor in women forming a negative perception of their birth in the long term (Waldenstrom et al 2004, Baston et al 2008, Rijnders et al 2008).

Midwives are often providing intimate physical and psychosocial care for women they have never met. Thus, student midwives who aim to provide effective midwifery care need to develop the ability to listen to the woman, to develop a relationship that demonstrates respect for her as an individual and to show understanding of her unique needs. The student midwife is potentially a great asset to the labouring woman. She can provide continuous support in a situation where the mentoring midwife may be caring for other women simultaneously. However, in order to provide effective care the student must feel that she, too, is being supported. She should be able to ask questions without feeling stupid, and to question respectfully care that does not appear to reflect what the evidence suggests to be best practice.

The birth partner

The woman's partner (if she has one) should be encouraged to be actively involved in supporting the woman, if this is what she wants. In a study designed to measure fathers' attitudes and needs in relation to being with their partner during labour and birth (Hollins Martin 2008) it was identified that the majority of fathers wanted to be actively involved and considered themselves to be the most appropriate person to support their partner. However, some people feel anxious when confronted with a hospital environment and the unpredictability of labour. The midwife can help create a relaxed and friendly atmosphere by remaining calm and approachable and engaging with the father throughout labour (Fathers Direct 2007).

The partner may need some direction and praise themselves, in order to continue to provide support to the labouring woman. Practical support is valued by women (Ip 2000) and he or she may feel most useful if given an active role to play, such as massage and passing drinks, etc. The partner also needs to be valued as the person who knows the woman better than anyone else in the room.

Activity

Make sure you know what a Doula is. Find out if there is a written guideline in your maternity unit about who the woman may be supported by during labour.

Find out who is responsible for continuing to provide care for a woman who had planned to have a home birth but who has required hospital admission during labour.

Interprofessional working

Staff of all disciplines need to work together with the single aim of ensuring an optimum outcome for the woman and her baby:

While a pleasant environment is an important element in creating the right atmosphere, attitude of staff is of greater value.

(RCOG 2002:09)

Successive Confidential Enquiries into Maternal Deaths (Lewis 2004, 2007) highlight lack of communication and teamwork as significant contributory factors. Mutual respect between all professions is vital, not only to enable midwives to undertake their roles without unnecessary interference but also to know that when assistance is requested it is available and justified. While acknowledging that midwives are the key providers during labour, Porter (2003) underlines the principle that midwives must remain alert to deviation from a normal course and be prepared to take appropriate action. The midwife must refer to an appropriate health professional if she detects a deviation from normal that is outside her current sphere of practice (NMC 2004).

Maternal wellbeing

Nutrition

The practice of restricting women's oral intake during labour has been widespread although variable throughout the UK (Singata & Tranmer 2003). This tradition was based on the risk of aspiration of gastric contents during general anaesthesia, a potentially fatal complication. However, this risk has been significantly reduced due to more advanced anaesthetic techniques and preference for regional anaesthesia. Withholding fluids and food does not ensure an empty stomach (O'Sullivan 1994) but does increase the risk of ketosis during labour, especially in primiparous women (Broach & Newton 1988). Anderson (1998) challenges the concept that ketosis in labour is pathological, suggesting that it is a physiological response that does not require treatment. A small randomized controlled trial (Scrutton et al 1999) found that eating a light diet during labour prevented the development of ketosis but that residual gastric volume increased. Enkin et al (2000) suggests that a small, low-residue diet is a sensible alternative to fasting. As labour progresses, women are less inclined to eat, but will need to have regular fluid, determined by their thirst. NICE intrapartum guidelines (2007) support the intake of a light diet and oral fluid intake throughout labour. Care must also be taken to ensure that the woman does not force herself to consume excessive amounts of water over and above her thirst. Although few in number, there are cases reported in the literature where women and their babies have suffered serious complications caused by water intoxication during labour (Johansson et al 2002). NICE guidelines (2007) suggest that isotonic drinks may be more beneficial than water during established labour.

There is no evidence to support the use of antacids or H2-receptor antagonists routinely for low risk women in labour (NICE 2007). However, the use of opioids during labour is associated with delayed gastric motility (Jordan 2002), and the woman should not be encouraged to eat if she has received such pharmacological analgesia, either by the intramuscular or epidural route

(NICE 2007): the use of antacids or H2-receptor antagonists should be considered in this situation.

Activity

Find out why pregnant women are more at risk of Mendelson's syndrome.
Identify examples of food and drink that would be suitable for intake during early labour.

Bladder care

During labour it is advisable that the urinary bladder is emptied regularly. There are three main reasons for encouraging women to pass urine at least every 2 hours:

1. It serves as an excellent distraction, to pass some time and take a short walk
2. A full bladder can impede descent of the presenting part
3. Urine can be tested for the presence of protein and ketones, if appropriate.

Observations

Observations and care provided are written on a large document called a partogram. This provides a visual representation of how the labour is progressing as well as a summary of any drugs and/or care that has been administered. Where there are no

maternal or fetal risk factors, basic observations can be limited to (NICE 2007:27):

- Blood pressure 4-hourly
- Temperature 4-hourly
- Pulse hourly.

Any detected abnormality should be documented, reported to a senior midwife and lead to a change in the plan of care, with clear parameters of when to take further action.

Monitoring progress in labour

As labour advances, uterine contractions become more frequent, more painful and last longer. The woman will require more support and encouragement as the length of time between contractions reduces and they are more challenging to endure. Staying with the woman will enable the student to develop the essential midwifery skills of assessing the length, strength and frequency of contractions (with a gentle hand on the uterine fundus) and how they impact on the woman's behaviour. The frequency of contractions should be documented half-hourly (NICE 2007). Translating what she sees and feels to the partogram, as with all skills, gets easier with practice.

Vaginal examination is also employed to assess progress of labour, but should be limited in its use. NICE intrapartum care guidelines recommend vaginal examination every 4 hours, or more frequently in response to clinical circumstances or the woman's request. It should always be preceded by abdominal palpation to identify fetal lie, presentation and engagement, position and fetal heart rhythm. For procedure for vaginal examination, see Chapter 2.

The most important reason for vaginal examination should be to provide feedback to the woman about how her labour is progressing. She should always be the first to know what the findings are – it is her information. Other indications sometimes used include: to confirm presentation; to exclude cord prolapse following rupture of the membranes; to rupture the forewaters; to prepare for administration of pharmacological pain relief; to confirm full dilation; and/or to apply fetal scalp electrode. Many of these indications are of doubtful necessity (Hanson 2003), and should not be used as an opportunity 'just to see what is happening'. Midwives should also tune in to the other signs that labour is progressing well and not rely too heavily on this invasive examination for her information (Hoadley 2007). As vaginal examination is an imprecise tool when conducted by different practitioners, where possible the same midwife should undertake subsequent examinations.

A midwife should supervise students undertaking vaginal examination so that she can describe her findings and receive guidance and instruction. This procedure can be uncomfortable and embarrassing for women, and it is all too easy for the student who is endeavouring to interpret what she is feeling to neglect the fact that there is a thinking, feeling women attached to the cervix she is trying to find.

The findings from abdominal palpation and vaginal examination should be written on the partogram. This tool alerts the practitioner if progress in active labour falls outside cervical dilatation of 1 cm an hour. Following a large randomized controlled trial (WHO 1994) it is recommended that *action* for delay in labour should only be taken if progress falls 4 cm to the right of the alert line, as this results in fewer caesarean births, less augmentation of labour and a reduced incidence of prolonged labour. A subsequent trial (Lavender et al 2006) confirmed that taking action after 2 hours increased intervention rates without improving maternal or neonatal outcomes, when compared to a 3- or 4-hour action line. NICE (2007) recommend the use of a 4-hour action line. See Box 3.1 for a summary of observations during the first stage of labour.

Fetal wellbeing

Amniotomy

Artificial rupture of the membranes (ARM), or amniotomy, is often performed under the pretext of establishing the condition of the liquor: is it meconium-stained or clear? In a large retrospective review, Eogan et al (2003) found that female infants were significantly more likely to have

Box 3.1 Summary of observations during the first stage of labour

- Blood pressure 4-hourly
- Temperature 4-hourly
- Pulse hourly
- Frequency of uterine contraction half-hourly
- Fetal heart rate every 15 minutes, for one full minute
- Fetal movements
- Frequency of bladder emptying
- Examination of vaginal loss
- Abdominal palpation 4-hourly
- Vaginal examination 4-hourly.

meconium-stained liquor. The incidence has also been seen to increase with gestational age (Wong et al 2002). When conducted in association with abnormalities of the fetal heart, the risks to the fetus are increased (Enkin et al 2000).

Amniotomy is also performed in order to shorten labour. However, in a systematic review of the evidence regarding the use of amniotomy to reduce the length of labour (Smyth et al 2007), there was no evidence that it achieved this aim and some evidence that it increased the risk of caesarean birth. The reviewers concluded that it should not be used for labours that are progressing normally or slowly. ARM is also associated with a sudden increase in the intensity of contractions, making them more difficult to cope with. When amniotomy is indicated, it should only be performed following discussion with the woman prior to the vaginal examination.

Activity

Find out about amnio-infusion and the risks and benefits associated with this procedure.

Make sure you understand the function of the amniotic fluid.

Think about the risks associated with meconium-stained liquor.

Fetal heart rate monitoring

Electronic fetal heart rate monitoring has become part of hospital midwifery care, and its use is widespread in the UK. Indiscriminate use has been associated with increases in instrumental delivery and caesarean section, without any benefit to long-term neonatal outcome (Enkin et al 2000). In a study exploring midwives attitudes to the use of the cardiotocograph machine (CTG), midwives rejected the notion that they had become dependent on it (Sinclair

2001). However, it does require knowledge, experience and a trained eye to interpret the print-out effectively, and failure to interpret it accurately is a major concern and contibutory factor to intrapartum stillbirth (CESDI 2000). It is a recommendation of the Clinical Negligence Scheme for Trusts that staff receive regular training in the interpretation of CTG traces.

In 2001, the National Institute for Clinical Excellence published guidelines that provide clear indications for electronic fetal monitoring in labour. Where no maternal or fetal risk factors are known, there is no need for an admission assessment (CTG) (Impey et al 2003) or continuous monitoring (Alfirevic et al 2006) and this stance has been reflected in further guidelines (NICE 2007). During the first stage of labour, the fetal heart should be auscultated after a contraction, for a full minute every 15 minutes. The fetal heart rate should be between 110 and 160 beats per minute.

Activity

List the indications for continuous electronic fetal monitoring.

Find out how often midwives are updated on the use and interpretation of CTG in the unit where you work.

Fetal movement

The fetus should remain active during labour. The midwife can use her enquiries about the baby's movements to motivate and encourage the woman to focus on her baby, to see her pain as having a purpose and that she will soon see the person she has so carefully nurtured.

Record-keeping

This aspect of the midwife's role is particularly challenging while caring for a woman in labour. The partogram provides an instant visual display of the care the woman has received and her progress in labour. It must be kept up-to-date so that if the woman requires any additional care while her primary carer, the midwife, is out of the room, it can be consulted and assumed to be a true record of recent events.

However, to be with a woman in active labour, rubbing her back and helping her with her breathing, is a full-time job. Opportunities can be snatched in between contractions to document key observations and events, but it can be particularly difficult to do so when something unexpected happens. The student midwife needs to develop the skill of noting the time of key events and creating a record that is clear and legible, dated, timed and signed. But this activity, although important, should not take the place of face-to-face interaction with the woman.

Records can and should be completed with the woman. It is information about her, information that is not 'just for the record' but which needs conveying to her in a way that is meaningful (and not at the height of a contraction).

In an emergency, the records should be completed as soon as possible after the event, and include precise details about who was called, when they attended and what action was planned as a result. Imagine the scenario. Fifteen years from now you are asked to describe the sequence of events that happened during a woman's labour. You only have the records you kept on that busy night to help you. Even if you felt sure that you had informed the doctor as soon as the fetal bradycardia was detected, unless the records state that you did and what the response had been it would be impossible to prove. A clear, detailed record is not only a tool for effective care but should be an honest portrayal of all key events.

Reflection on trigger

Look back on the trigger scenario.

Chloe had been experiencing painful uterine contractions for 10 hours with her first baby. She had been in hospital for 6 hours, and the midwife who had been caring for her was now going off duty. The midwife had handed over Chloe's care to a midwife who would also be looking after another woman in early labour. The midwife entered the room and said, 'Hello, I'm Margaret, I'm just going to put you on the monitor.'

Now that you are familiar with care of the woman during the first stage of labour you should have insight into how the scenario relates to this aspect of the midwife's role. The jigsaw model will now be used to explore the trigger scenario in more depth.

Effective communication

During the first stage of labour the woman and her partner will require feedback from the midwife about her progress and the wellbeing of her baby. In addition, the labour ward coordinator will need to be kept appraised of her progress so that she can provide appropriate support and guidance if necessary. Additionally, midwives handing over care need to ensure that they provide the incoming midwife with a detailed summary of the woman's history and current situation. Questions that arise from the scenario might include: How had the two midwives communicated about Chloe's labour progress? What opportunities are there for Chloe to communicate her aspirations for the birth? How does Margaret enable the woman to inform her if her needs change during labour? What systems are in place to enable Margaret to keep the labour ward coordinator informed of the woman's progress? How might you first address a woman that you meet for the first time in active labour?

Woman-centred care

During her labour the woman should be the central focus. She should be involved in all decsions about her care and feel that her views and wishes are respected. Questions that arise from the scenario might include: Does Margaret know how Chloe feels about having electronic fetal monitoring (EFM)? How does Margaret encourage Chloe to express her particular wishes regarding her labour? In what situations is woman-centred care compromised in the maternity unit? How might labouring at home have enhanced Chloe's sense that she is the focus of care? How often are midwives where you work also caring for another woman in labour?

Using best evidence

There is a range of research evidence to support the midwifery practices undertaken during the first stage of labour. However there are many aspects of care that midwives undertake because they have personal experience regarding their effectiveness. Questions that arise from the scenario might include: What evidence is informing Margaret's intention to commence electronic fetal monitoring? How does Margaret keep up-to-date with current research evidence? How has research informed Chloe's preparation for childbirth? How do women access sources of information about labour and birth? How will Chloe's experience of this birth inform any future birth aspirations? Has Chloe been exposed to birthing stories from her friends or relatives?

Professional and legal issues

It is part of the midwife's role to 'care for and assist the mother during labour and to monitor the condition of the fetus in utero by the appropriate clinical and technical means' (NMC 2004:37). The midwife is also required to 'ensure that you gain consent before you begin any treatment or care' (NMC 2008:04). Questions that arise from the scenario might include: Did Margaret seek or gain informed consent to commence EFM? If the labour ward policy required Margaret to monitor Chloe's labour electronically, what would Margaret need to do if Chloe declined this intervention? What alternative clinical means could Margaret use to monitor the wellbeing of Chloe and her baby?

Team working

The midwife does not work in isolation but as part of the larger multidiciplinary team. As a registered practitioner, the midwife must ensure that she 'consults and takes advice from colleagues when appropriate' (NMC 2008:05). Questions that arise from the scenario might include: What is the role of the labour ward coordinator and in what circumstances should their advice be sought? When might Margaret refer Chloe to a medical practitioner during the first stage of labour? Which other health workers support the care of women in labour either directly or indirectly? How can Margaret involve Chloe's partner in her care? When is it appropriate to discuss a woman's progress with her birth partner?

Clinical dexterity

The student midwife must develop a range of clinical skills in order to provide safe and effective care to women during the first stage of labour. She will learn some of these in the safe environment of the Clinical Simulation Unit at University but will practice, enhance and maintain them whilst providing clinical care to women.

Questions that arise from the scenario might include: What skills are required to monitor Chloe's progress in labour? How did Margaret acquire and develop them? How is clinical competence assessed at the point of registration? Does Chloe have a student caring for her? If so, how will this impact on her experience of labour? In what circumstances should a student not duplicate care with the sole aim of enhancing her clinical dexterity?

Models of care

The model of care that women choose for labour and birth will have a significant influence on the way that care is provided. Women who come into hospital to birth their babies have access to a range of interventions designed to monitor, mitigate or manage their labours. Questions that arise from the scenario might include: How might Chloe's experience of the first stage of labour have been different if she had stayed at home or accessed a home from home unit? Was Chloe offered an alternative model of care? What are the advantages and disadvantages of labouring in hospital? Will Margaret be able to provide one-to-one support for Chloe during her labour? Will Chloe be left alone at a time when it worries her to be without professional contact?

Safe environment

Midwives are required to provide safe and effective clinical care and in so doing must ensure that the environment in which they work does not expose

women to unnecessary risk. Labour wards are often very busy places to work in, accessed by a range of personnel and home to a plethora of complex equipment requiring close supervision and careful maintenance. Questions that arise from the scenario might include: Is the electronic fetal monitor that Margaret is hoping to use maintained in line with the manufacturer's guidelines? Have the transducers' belts been changed in between clients? How are the transducers cleaned in between women? When did Margaret last update her skills in interpreting fetal heart rate traces? Are there sufficient midwives on duty to respond to suspected fetal compromise?

Promotes health

Ensuring that the woman maintains good health throughout her labour is an aim of the surveillance and care activities the midwife undertakes. The midwife must ensure that the woman remains well hydrated and receives sufficient nourishment to meet the challenges posed by labour and birth. The midwife must monitor the woman's skin integrity, facilitate her elimination requirements and help her find appropriate strategies to deal with regular uterine contractions. Questions that arise from the scenario might include: How might the use of EFM hinder Chloe's coping strategies? What strategies can Margaret employ to help maximize the chances of Chloe having a spontaneous vaginal birth? How can Margaret help Chloe have a positive birth experience?

Further scenarios

The following scenarios enable you to consider how specific situations influence the care the midwife provides. Use the jigsaw model to explore the issues raised in the scenario.

Scenario 1

Kirsty is 17 and is admitted to the labour ward with strong uterine contractions every 3 minutes. She is accompanied by her mother and her boyfriend. Kirsty's mother does all the talking, her boyfriend appears very shy and stands away from Kirsty.

Practice point

It is not possible to dictate or stipulate who is the best person to accompany a woman in labour. Some women have attended childbirth preparation classes with their partner and/or have discussed how they wish to be supported in labour. Others wish their mother or sister to support them but want the father to be present in the hope that it will help facilitate them in their future role: most fathers also believe that this is the best start to fatherhood (Hollins Martin 2008). Some women may hope that their partner will be supportive but in the event find that the environment is alienating or the circumstances overwhelming. For some women, it is appropriate that they have more than one person to provide support in different ways. Young fathers usually want to be involved but sometimes feel unwelcome (Fathers Direct 2007).

Further questions specific to Scenario 1 include:

1. Is the boyfriend the father of the baby?
2. How can the midwife enable the boyfriend to support Kirsty?
3. Does Kirsty want her boyfriend to support her?
4. Does Kirsty's boyfriend want to actively support her?
5. Does Kirsty want both of them to stay throughout labour?
6. What facilities are there to accommodate birth attendants?

Scenario 2

Jenny is planning to have her baby at home. She is in active labour and two midwives are sitting in the kitchen. Jenny comes through from the next door room and says, 'Phew, that last contraction was a whopper!' She then asks them if they want a cup of tea.

Practice point

Staying at home during labour can help the woman feel relaxed and enjoy labour, confident in her surroundings and support networks. The midwife remains a guest in the woman's home and the woman should be able to maintain control of when she eats, drinks and goes to the toilet. She is free to roam around without needing to ask permission.

Further questions specific to Scenario 2 include:

1. Have the midwives discussed with Jenny if she wants them in the same

room as her during the first stage of labour?

2. Should the midwives accept Jenny's offer of a cup of tea and/or offer to make it for her?

3. Where is the student midwife?

4. Who else is supporting Jenny throughout her labour?

5. Has Jenny previously met the midwives who have come to care for her?

6. What happens if Jenny's labour goes beyond the midwives shift?

Conclusion

Student midwives have a significant role to play in providing support and effective care to labouring women. Being 'with woman' enables the development of a trusting and respectful relationship. Providing continuous presence and active engagement will contribute to an optimum outcome for all involved.

Resources

ABC of Labour Care: British Medical Journal. Useful diagrams. http://www.bmj.com/cgi/content/full/318/7186/793.

Association of Radical Midwives: Artificial rupture of membranes. http://www.radmid.demon.co.uk/arm.htm.

Indexed visuals: Normal vaginal birth animation. http://www.indexedvisuals.com/scripts/ivstock/pic.asp?id=130N-299.

NHS Direct: Information for patients: labour. http://www.prodigy.nhs.uk/patient_information_leaflet/labour#339229000.

References

Alfirevic Z, Devane D, Gyte GML: Continuous cardiotocography (CTG) as a form of electronic fetal monitoring (EFM) for fetal assessment during labour DOI: 10.1002/14651858. CD006066, *Cochrane Database of Systematic Reviews* 3(CD006066), 2006.

Anderson T: Is ketosis in labour pathological?, *The Practising Midwife* 1(9):22–26, 1998.

Baston H, Rijnders M, Green J, et al: Looking back on birth 3 years later: factors associated with a negative appraisal in England and in the Netherlands, *Journal of Reproductive & Infant Psychology* 26(4):323–339, 2008.

Berg M, Lundgren I, Hermansson E, et al: Women's experience of the encounter with the midwife during childbirth, *Midwifery* 12:11–15, 1996.

Broach J, Newton N: Food and beverages in labor. Part II: the effects of cessation of oral intake during labor, *Birth* 15(2):88–92, 1988.

CESDI: Confidential enquiry into stillbirths and deaths in infancy: *7th Annual Report*, London, 2000, Maternal and Child Health Consortium.

Commission for Healthcare Audit and Inspection: *Women's experiences of maternity care in the NHS in England*, London, 2007, Healthcare Commission.

Department of Health: *Making it better: for mother and baby. Clinical case for change (Shribman)*, London, 2007a, Department of Health.

Department of Health: *Maternity matters: choice, access and continuity of care in a safe service*, London, 2007b, Department of Health.

Enkin M, Keirse M, Neilson J, et al: *A guide to effective care in pregnancy and childbirth*, ed 3, Oxford, 2000, Oxford University Press.

Eogan M, Geary M, O'Connell M, et al: Effect of fetal sex on labour and delivery: retrospective review, *British Medical Journal* 326:137, 2003.

Fathers Direct: Including new fathers. A guide for maternity professionals, 2007. Online. Available www.fathersdirect. com July 31, 2008.

Green J, Coupland V, Kitzinger J: *Great expectations. A prospective study of women's expectations and experiences of childbirth*, Hale, 1998, Books for Midwives Press.

Green J, Baston H: Feeling in control during labour: concepts, correlates and consequences, *Birth* 30(4):235–247, 2003.

Green J, Baston H: Greater expectations? A prospective study of expectations and experiences of

intrapartum care in 1987 and 2000. *Book of Abstracts presented at the XIV International Congress of ISPOG, Edinburgh, Scotland*, May 16–19. Oxon, 2004, Parthenon Publishing, 25:125.

Hanson S: To VE or not VE? That is the question, *Midwifery Matters* 97:16–17, 2003.

Hoadley J: Assessing progress in labour: midwife and woman in partnership, *MIDIRS Midwifery Digest* 17(1):75–77, 2007.

Hodnett ED, Downe S, Edwards N, et al: Home-like versus conventional institutional settings for birth DOI: 10.1002/14651858.CD000012.pub2, *Cochrane Database of Systematic Reviews* 4(CD000012), 2004.

Hodnett ED, Gates S, Hofmeyr GJ, et al: Continuous support for women during childbirth DOI: 10.1002/14651858.CD003766.pub2, *Cochrane Database of Systematic Reviews* 2(CD003766), 2007.

Hollins Martin C: A tool to measure fathers' attitudes and needs in relation to birth, *British Journal of Midwifery* 16(7):432–437, 2008.

Impey L, Reynolds M, Macquillan K, et al: Admission cardiotocography: a randomised controlled trial, *The Lancet* 361:465–470, 2003.

Ip W: Relationship between partner's support during labour and maternal outcomes, *Journal of Clinical Nursing* 9:265–272, 2000.

Johansson S, Lindow S, Kapadia H, et al: Perinatal water intoxication due to excessive oral intake during labour, *Acta Paediatrica* 91(7):811–814, 2002.

Jordan S: *Pharmacology for midwives: the evidence base for safe practice*, Basingstoke, 2002, Palgrave.

King's Fund: *Safe Birth: everybody's business. An independent inquiry into the safety of maternity services in England*, London, 2008, King's Fund.

Lavender T, Alfirevic Z, Walkinshaw SA: Effect of different action lines on birth outcomes: a randomized controlled trial, *Obstetrics & Gynecology* 108(2):295–302, 2006.

Lewis G, editor: Confidential enquiries into maternal and child health. Why mothers die. *The sixth report of the United Kingdom confidential enquiries into maternal deaths in the United Kingdom,* London, 2004, RCOG Press.

Lewis GE: The confidential enquiry into maternal and child health (CEMACH). Saving mothers' lives: reviewing maternal deaths to make motherhood safer – 2003–2005. The seventh report on confidential enquiries into maternal deaths in the United Kingdom, London, 2007, CEMACH.

Maternity Care Working Party: *Making normal birth a reality. Consensus statement from the Maternity Care Working Party (MCWP)*, London, 2007, Maternity Care Working Party.

Newburn M: Culture, control and the birth environment, *The Practising Midwife* 6(8):20–25, 2003.

National Institute for Health and Clinical Excellence (NICE): *Intrapartum care. Care of healthy women and their babies during childbirth. NICE clinical guideline 55*, London, 2007, NICE.

Nursing and Midwifery Council (NMC): *Midwives rules and standards*, London, 2004, NMC.

Nursing and Midwifery Council (NMC): *The Code. Standards of conduct, performance and ethics for nurse and midwives*, London, 2008, NMC.

Osterman P, Schwartz-Barcott D: Presence: four ways of being there, *Nursing Forum* 31(2):23–30, 1996.

O'Sullivan G: The stomach: fact and fantasy. Eating and drinking during labour, *International Anesthesiology Clinics* 32:31–44, 1994.

Porter R: Expectations of the midwife's role: supporting normal birth, *MIDIRS Midwifery Digest* 13(2):217–219, 2003.

RCOG: *Clinical standards: advice on planning the service in obstetrics and gynaecology*, London, 2002, Royal College of Obstetricians and Gynaecologists.

Redshaw M, Rowe R, Hockley C, et al: *Recorded delivery: a national survey of women's experience of maternity care*, Oxford, 2007, National Perinatal Epidemiology Unit.

Rijnders M, Baston H, Schonbeck Y, et al: Perinatal factors related to a negative or positive recall of birth experience in women 3 years postpartum in the Netherlands, *Birth* 35(2):107–116, 2008.

Royal College of Obstetricians and Gynaecologists: *Standards for maternity* care. *Report of a working party*, London, 2008, RCOG.

Scrutton M, Metcalfe G, Lowy C, et al: Eating in labour. A randomised controlled trial assessing the risks and benefits, *Anaesthesia* 54(4):329–334, 1999.

Sinclair M: Midwives' attitudes to the use of the cardiotocograph machine, *Journal of Advanced Nursing* 35(4): 599–606, 2001.

Singata M, Tranmer J: *Restricting oral fluid and food intake during labour (protocol for a Cochrane Review)* The Cochrane Library, 4, Chichester, UK, 2003, John Wiley & Sons.

Smyth RMD, Alldred SK, Markham C: Amniotomy for shortening spontaneous labour DOI: 10.1002/14651858. CD006167.pub2, *Cochrane Database of Systematic Reviews* 4(CD006167), 2007.

Waldenstrom U, Hildingsson I, Rubertsson C, et al: A negative birth experience: prevalence and risk factors in a national sample, *Birth* 31(1):17–27, 2004.

Weaver J: Choice, control and decision-making in labour. In Clement S, editor: *Psychological persepectives on pregnancy and childbirth*, Edinburgh, 1998, Churchill Livingstone.

Wong S, Chow K, Ho L: The relative risk of 'fetal distress' in pregnancy associated with meconium-stained liquor at different gestations, *Journal of Obstetrics and Gynaecology* 22(6): 594–599, 2002.

World Health Organization: *The application of the WHO partograph in the management of labour* WHO/IHE/MSM 94.4, Geneva, 1994, WHO.

Chapter 4

Non-pharmacological methods of coping with labour

Trigger scenario

Leanne is in spontaneous labour with her second baby. She has just arrived on the hospital birth suite and is experiencing painful uterine contractions every 3 minutes. She is finding the pain in her lower back very difficult to cope with. Leanne had an epidural during her first labour and would like to try to manage without one this time.

Introduction

This chapter considers non-pharmacological methods of pain relief used during labour (pharmacological methods will be covered in Chapter 6). The woman's experience of pain in childbirth is unique to her (Waldenstrom et al 1996) and mediated by her previous experiences (Niven & Gijspers 1990),

and her social and cultural circumstances (Seymour 1997). For some women experiencing pain in labour is linked to their spiritual beliefs (Hall 2001, Walsh 2007, Hall & Taylor 2008). The link between a woman's expectations and experience of pain are linked with her level of satisfaction with labour and antenatal education regarding what to expect (Lally et al 2008).The individual needs of women vary and what works for one person may not suit the next. However, it is suggested that the attitudes of the birth attendants have an effect on what ways women choose in order to cope with pain of labour (Leap & Anderson 2008). They go on to write about different views of either wanting to relieve pain for women, or to want to help women 'work with' their pain, which is related to the caregivers' own attitudes and beliefs.

It is often remarked that the pain of labour is quickly forgotten, consumed by the joy associated with the safe arrival of the baby. However, in a review of the literature, Niven & Murphy-Black (2000) conclude that labour pain, although not always recalled with accuracy, is not completely forgotten. In a study asking women of their memory of pain 2 months and 1 year after the birth, 47% of women still remembered the same level of pain after 1 year, with 35% remembering the pain as less severe (Waldenstrom 2003). In order to help minimize the degree of pain experienced, the midwife will need a range of strategies that she can suggest and support the woman with. Women may also have their own ideas – perhaps passed on from other women or methods that they have previously used themselves (Spiby et al 2003).

Why is labour painful?

Box 4.1 shows the identified theories about the purpose of pain in labour (from Leap & Anderson 2008).

As labour progresses, so, too, does the length and duration of uterine contractions. In addition, the cervix dilates and the pelvic floor and vagina stretch as the presenting part of the fetus descends the birth canal. Thoracic, lumbar and sacral nerves transmit the resultant painful stimuli (Hamilton 2003). The balance of hormones, such as oxytocin, beta-endorphins and adrenaline, will also have an effect on the pain a woman experiences (Buckley 2005). Fear of labour appears to have a direct link to how women experience pain (Saisto 2001). What a woman may well have been coping with quite easily may become more and more difficult to endure.

Activity

Reflect on your first experience of physical pain.
What is the treatment you usually take for a common pain, for example, a headache? Why do you choose this form of pain relief?

Box 4.1: Theories about the purpose of pain in labour (from Leap Anderson 2008:41)

- Pain as pure psychology
- Pain stops women and allows them to find a place of safety to give birth
- Pain marks the occasion
- Pain summons support
- Pain develops altruistic behaviour towards babies
- Pain heightens joy
- Pain is the transition to motherhood
- Pain gives clues to progress
- Pain reinforces the triumph of going through labour
- Pain is a trigger of neurohormonal cascades.

Non-pharmacological methods

Women have always sought to cope with their labour pain by using a range of behaviours and practices. The use of pharmacological methods of pain relief is often associated with unwanted side-effects (Walsh 2007). Employing the use of non-pharmacological methods has the potential to delay (or prevent) the use of medication and the subsequent total dose received (Simkin & O'Hara 2002). A large prospective study (Green 1993) found that women who avoided the use of medication were also more likely to be satisfied with the birth than those who used drugs. Women who want to keep drug use to a minimum during labour are more likely to do so (Green et al 1998), as are those who have confidence in their ability to cope or 'self-efficacy' for labour (Lowe 1989).

One of the important features of non-pharmacological methods of coping in the early stages of labour is distraction. Later in labour women may need to 'go into themsleves' (Thompson 2004:33) and not be disturbed

(Odent 2002). Each time another strategy is employed, time has moved on and, hopefully, so has the labour. They must, however, be significant, appropriate, realistic strategies, as the woman will soon grow to distrust the midwife's judgment if she suggests the impossible. The concept of 'working with the pain' (Leap & Anderson 2008) demonstrates that the process is active and not passive. Non-pharmacological techniques often involve the continued presence of a midwife or birth partner, which has been shown to reduce the need for pharmacological methods of pain relief (Hodnett et al 2007).

Although this chapter focuses on non-pharmacological methods, in practice women will often combine these with pharmacological methods to achieve a level of coping that meets their specific plans and needs. As methods such as breathing techniques also have the additional benefit of reducing panic and helping the woman to stay calm, such methods should be encouraged throughout labour if pharmacological methods are also employed (Spiby et al 2003).

Role of the midwife

The midwife caring for a woman in labour needs to establish if the woman has expectations and plans regarding how to cope with labour. She should consult her birth plan (if there is one) and, in discussion with her, explore the most appropriate course of action. There should be mutual acknowledgement that this plan is flexible and may need to adapt to changing needs and circumstances. No one can predict the precise course of any labour although, with experience and vigilant observation of the woman's behaviour, the midwife can provide useful feedback to the woman to help inform her decisions.

In a systematic review of the literature on pain and women's satisfaction with the experience, Hodnett (2002) concluded that the amount of support from caregivers and involvement in decision-making are more important contributors to satisfaction than childbirth preparation, continuity of care and pain. As a midwife, it is part of your role to provide care and support to women in labour (NMC 2004) based on current evidence (NMC 2007a). However, where a woman requires specific intervention that is outside your sphere of practice, you must acknowledge the limits of your current competence.

The Rules and Standards for Midwives [6.3] state if a situation arises for a midwife:

which is outside her current sphere of practice becomes apparent in a woman or baby during the antenatal, intranatal or postnatal periods, a practising midwife shall call such qualified health professionals as may reasonably be expected to have the necessary skills and experience to assist her in the provision of care

(NMC 2004:08)

Parity

It is worth noting that, although generally speaking, second and subsequent labours are shorter than those of primigravida, the speed and intensity of progress can suddenly overwhelm a multiparous woman. She may have had an epidural with her first labour and be fearful of feeling the actual birth. She will need just as much support and reassurance as a primigravida, and acknowledgement of her previous experiences.

Labouring in water

Pain in labour can lead to tension and fear. Warm water helps release muscle tension and promote a sense of general wellbeing. The use of the bath in labour has the additional benefit of enabling women to feel more in control (Hall & Holloway 1998) and experience less pain (Cluett et al 2002, Eberhard et al 2005). However, bathing before labour is established may lead to contractions slowing down. Michel Odent (2002:109) recommends the use of showers prior to getting into the bath or pool. In a systematic review of the evidence, Simkin & O'Hara (2002) conclude that the woman should be in established labour before immersion in water and that it should not last more than 1–2 hours (although it can be returned to later in labour). The activity of getting in and out of the pool may be beneficial in establishing the pattern of the labour.

Women may worry that bathing after their membranes have ruptured might be contraindicated. Bathing following ruptured membranes is not associated with increased infection rates (Eriksson et al 1996). However, prolonged exposure to hot bath water may result in a rise in fetal temperature and heart rate. Anderson (2004) suggested that the women themselves should be able to monitor the most appropriate temperature for the water. However it is advised that maternal temperature and the fetal heart rate should be closely observed during hot water immersion and the temperature of the water should not be above 37.5°C (NICE 2007). See Chapter 5 for further detail regarding use of water in labour.

Breathing techniques

As we go about our everyday lives, we pay little attention to our breathing patterns. Breathing is usually effortless, nasal breathing with a natural pause following expiration. When we experience pain, however, our breathing becomes shallower and more rapid and the 'gap' is lost. When in severe pain, we hold our breath as our face grimaces.

The role of the midwife and supporters in labour is to notice when the woman changes her breathing pattern and to encourage her back to

as near normal breathing as possible. Although the woman may have had the opportunity to practise breathing techniques antenatally, this is not essential and midwives can guide her in this if required, enabling the woman to relax and regain control. One technique may be:

Sitting facing her, at eye level, ask her to copy you. Breathe in through your nose and very gently and slowly, blow out through your mouth. This may be less helpful at the times when a woman has 'gone into herself' as described above (Thompson 2004:33). The more advanced the labour, the more rapid her breathing will become, but she will need encouragement to slow her breathing down to avoid the light-headedness caused by hyperventilation. Her birth partner may also be involved in this role as s/he can keep the woman focused if the midwife needs to leave the room.

In a prospective study of women's expectations and experiences in labour (Green at al 1998), women who expected breathing and relaxation to be useful antenatally were more likely to report that they had been, when surveyed 6 weeks after the birth.

Activity

Not only does activity during labour serve to distract from the focus on each moment of each contraction, but it enables the body to work with gravity as the fetus negotiates its way into the pelvis. Women who remain upright during labour report less severe pain (de Jong et al 1999). Activity during the first stage of labour has also been shown to reduce its mean duration for both primigravida and multigravida by 3 and 2 hours respectively (Allahbadia & Vaidya 1992).

Activity is ideally suited for the home environment, where women can move from room to room, using familiar furniture to lean against during contractions. Once in hospital, the bed is often the central feature of the birthing room. Women may need encouragement to get up from it following an abdominal or vaginal examination, and to use the room as their own, moving freely around it. Although birth rooms are often designed with the attendants and equipment in mind rather than freedom of movement for the woman, it is often possible to create a more comfortable environment by removing superfluous equipment, pushing a bed to one side and bringing in accessories such as a beanbag or ball.

Disability

Midwives need to work in partnership with women with disability to meet their individual needs (Bowler 2008). There is a range of equipment available to enable women with a disability to maintain independence during labour (Brown & Brown 2003). For example, most maternity units have some birthing beds that can be controlled electronically, enabling the woman to alter its height or the position of the backrest without assistance.

Complementary and alternative therapies

There are many therapies used by midwives across the world, ranging from simple massage to bioelectric or magnetic applications (Allaire et al 2000, Walsh 2007). The four most commonly offered in maternity services in the UK are massage, aromatherapy, reflexology and acupuncture (Mitchell et al 2006). Tritten (2002) argues that midwives must respect and learn from traditional midwives and healers before the knowledge base is lost.

Although complementary therapies are not generally part of the midwifery curriculum, the University of the West of England (UWE) has developed and implemented a module into its midwifery programme (Mitchell & Doyle 2002). Evaluation has shown that students have found the module useful and relevant, although some have been frustrated by its varied acceptance by qualified midwives working in acute settings.

All therapies, however, must be provided by skilled and competent practitioners, and only given with the woman's informed consent (NMC 2004, Tiran 2007). Fundamental to the administration of medication by a midwife is Rule 7 which states:

A practising midwife shall only supply and administer those medicines, including analgesics, in respect of which she has received the appropriate training as to use, dosage and methods of administration.

(NMC 2004:19)

This clear guidance also applies to the use of homeopathic substances, although the woman's right to self-administer such remedies must be respected. Midwives need to be aware that a woman may be using therapies routinely, as part of her life, and that these may not be appropriate during pregnancy.

Activity

Find out if women where you work are routinely asked if they currently use or aim to use complementary therapies.

Investigate whether there is a local policy for the use of complementary therapies in labour.

There are many alternative therapies that can be used by labouring women. This chapter will focus on massage, aromatherapy, and acupuncture as methods that are increasingly being used.

Massage

The use of touch and massage during labour conveys encouragement and concern (Chang et al 2002). Massage can involve the use of an inert base oil with or without the addition of essential oils.

A randomized controlled trial found that women reported significant emotional and physical relief from massage by their partners (Field et al 1997). However, for some women being touched in labour may be inappropriate and it is important to communicate about this in preparation for labour as well as asking permission beforehand (Kitzinger 1997). Massage can also be used in conjunction with other strategies and is an ideal way of involving the birth partner in supportive care of the labouring women. Kimber (2002) describes an antenatal programme in Banbury for couples, which combines massage with breathing techniques and visualization. However, a recent pilot randomized controlled trial has identified that massage alone may provide relief of pain (Kimber et al 2008).

Aromatherapy

Aromatherapy is 'the art and science of using essential plant oils in treatment' (Davis 1991:01). The use of aromatherapy appears to be developing more commonly as a practice (Mitchell et al 2006). Supported by evidence-based guidelines, midwives who have undertaken further education and assessment of competence administer a selection of essential oils to women during labour and postnatally (Dhany 2008). This service is also available to women having a home birth, and audit of the service has shown that women generally find aromatherapy helpful, although there is insufficient trial evidence about its effectiveness (Smith et al 2006).

Acupuncture

Acupuncture involves the insertion of sterile acupuncture needles at specific acupuncture points. Needling of some points invokes relaxation, whereas others produce an analgesic effect. Needles can be taped in place to allow freedom of movement. A randomized controlled trial of acupuncture during labour (Ramnero et al 2002) found that women in the experimental group were significantly less likely to need an epidural (12% versus 22% in the control group). However, there was no difference between the groups with regard to mean pain intensity. A meta-analysis of seven trials (Smith et al 2006) reported significantly more relaxation in the acupuncture group than the control group. The NICE Intrapartum Care Guidelines (2007) do not recommend the use of acupuncture in labour but that women should not be stopped from using it if they wish.

Transcutaneous electrical nerve stimulation (TENS)

TENS comprises a small operating unit (about the size of a portable radio) and four thin leads connected to sticky pads (electrodes). These are applied to specific acupuncture pressure points on the back, delivering a pulsed electrical current to the surface of the skin (Fig. 4.1). The unit is battery operated and can be attached to a belt. The woman uses a hand-held device to boost the current during contractions.

TENS is thought to work by stimulating the release of endorphins and by blocking the transmission of pain impulses to the brain. A systematic review (Carroll et al 1997) concluded that there was no substantial evidence for TENS having an analgesic effect during labour, although the use of additional methods of pain relief may be reduced. The placebo effect may be of value, however: in a study comparing TENS with placebo TENS, both groups reported a reduction in pain, although there were no significant differences between them (van der Ploeg et al 1996). The evidence shows that the use of TENS in established labour is not effective and therefore its use is not recommended (NICE 2007). Availability of TENS machines varies between maternity units, although there are many companies that hire or sell them, including high street stores.

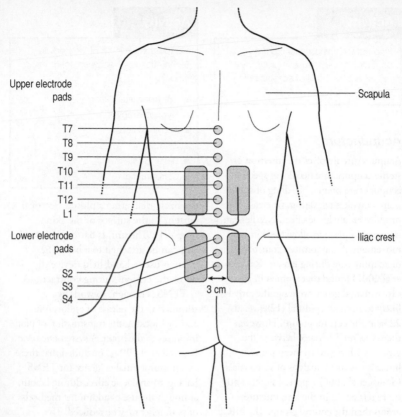

Upper electrode pads

Scapula

T7
T8
T9
T10
T11
T12
L1

Lower electrode pads

Iliac crest

S2
S3
S4

3 cm

Fig. 4.1 Positioning for TENS electrodes. (Adapted with kind permission from Coates 1998.)

Record-keeping

This is an essential part of the midwife's role, and particularly so when caring for a woman in labour. Your records must demonstrate that you have assessed her condition and discussed the options available to her in the context of her progress in labour. You must then document what care has been provided and evaluate the impact of your actions. So, for example, if the woman decides to try a warm bath because she has backache, the records should describe when she entered the water and how successful the bath was in alleviating her pain (in addition to the continuing assessment of maternal and fetal wellbeing during active labour). If the bath did not help, the records should include what further action was taken, following discussions with the woman.

If the woman decides on a course of action that you feel could jeopardize either maternal or fetal wellbeing, despite providing her with a clear rationale for your concern, you must inform a senior midwife and document your discussion, while continuing to provide care and support. The development of a trusting, respectful relationship at the onset of your contact will make continued dialogue more likely. You must remember that the woman has the right to read her records and they should be written in a non-judgmental, clear and factual manner (NMC 2007b).

Reflection on trigger

Look back on the trigger scenario at the start of the chapter.

Leanne is in spontaneous labour with her second baby. She has just arrived on the hospital birth suite and is experiencing painful uterine contractions every 3 minutes. She is finding the pain in her lower back very difficult to cope with. Leanne had an epidural during her first labour and would like to try to manage without one this time.

The scenario is one that any hospital-based midwife could face on a daily basis. It raises issues relating to communication about Leanne's past history, as well as her

present desires and choices for this labour. Now that you are familiar with the use of methods of coping in labour you should have insight into how the scenario relates to the evidence. The jigsaw model will now be used to explore the trigger scenario in more depth.

Effective communication

In this situation Leanne may not have met the midwife before. Therefore there is a need to build up a relationship quickly, so that Leanne feels safe and trusts the midwife in this situation. Questions that could be asked include: How will the midwife greet Leanne to make her feel welcome and more at ease? What questions will need to be asked about Leanne's previous experience? What questions will need to be asked about strategies Leanne has already used at home? Has she written a birth plan? What questions will need to be asked about strategies Leanne wishes to use for this labour?

Woman-centred care

In order to provide woman-centred care for Leanne the midwife needs to establish what her needs and wants are. This can be a challenge as Leanne is in labour and feeling pain. Questions that could be asked include: Has Leanne written a birth plan that could guide the midwife? What are her needs and desires at this moment of the labour? How can the midwife ensure Leanne remains central to the care during labour? How will she present choices to Leanne?

Using best evidence

In order to provide evidence-based care the midwife needs to be up-to-date with research evidence. However, she will also use evidence from her previous knowledge of caring for women in labour, as well as evidence from Leanne's background of how she coped in her previous labour. Questions that need to be addressed to ensure that the woman's care is evidence-based include: What is the evidence around helping women to cope in labour? As Leanne is experiencing pain in her back what could the midwife deduce from this evidence? What do the midwife's local guidelines say about pain strategies for labour? What evidence is this based on?

Professional and legal

The responsibilities of midwives in the UK regarding the use of methods of pain relief are covered by rules and codes (NMC 2004). Midwives should be appropriately trained in the use of particular methods on offer for women in labour and should be aware of who to contact for further support and advice. Questions that could be asked include: Has the midwife been trained in the use of methods of supporting pain prior to qualification? Has she required further training following qualification and is this up-to-date? What NMC rules or codes relate to these methods? How do the local guidelines or national guidelines relate to these methods?

Team working

In straightforward labour a midwife may care for a woman on her own.

However, a midwife usually works in a multidisciplinary setting, and may call on assistance as required. In this situation the midwife and Leanne will be working in partnership, alongside Leanne's birth supporter if she has one with her. The midwife will aim to establish the best strategies to help Leanne in labour. Questions that may be asked include: How may a midwife ensure team working with Leanne and her supporters? Will other people need to be informed of the strategies chosen? Has Leanne invited a complementary therapy practitioner to assist her from outside the NHS? How can the midwife work with this practitioner?

Clinical dexterity

In this situation the midwife may require dexterity in the strategies employed, particularly in the use of touch, massage and aromatherapy. Questions that may be asked include: Has the midwife been trained appropriately to be dextrous? Are there ways that she could practice some of these strategies in another situation? Does she need to carry out the strategy or can this be shown to the partner to do instead? How does Leanne feel about the strategies being employed?

Models of care

In the situation illustrated the midwife may not have had an opportunity to build up a relationship with Leanne prior to her coming to the birth suite. In other situations Leanne may have had the opportunity to get to know her midwife over pregnancy and have her caring for her in labour. Questions that may be asked include: Does the model illustrated here impact on the way Leanne copes with labour? How can the midwife ensure that the fact they have not met does not hinder Leanne's care and perceptions of her experience? How does the environment support the use of complementary therapies?

Safe environment

In this situation the midwife needs to ensure the environment is the most appropriate in order to meet Leanne's needs. Questions that may be asked include: Will another room need to be prepared for the strategies to be employed? Is there anyone already in that room? When will it become available? Is the space adequate to enable Leanne to have safe ease of movement? If not, is there somewhere else available? Is the use of any of the strategies harmful to the midwife or other members of the team in that environment?

Promotes health

The use of non-pharmacological strategies may be less harmful to the unborn infant in the long term, but not if the experience causes the woman emotional trauma or distress. The midwife needs to balance all the issues that are affecting Leanne and her perceptions of the experience to ensure she remains empowered. Questions that may be asked include: What are the advantages of Leanne using these strategies to help her? Are any of the strategies used going to be harmful to her or her unborn baby?

Further scenarios

The following scenarios enable you to consider how specific situations influence the care the midwife provides. Use the jigsaw model to explore the issues raised in the scenario.

Scenario 1

Amanda receives a call at the birth unit. Verity is in labour with her first baby. According to her notes the baby is in a breech presentation. She has declined a caesarean section and would like to use the birth pool as a strategy for coping.

Practice point

Breech presentations are considered to be more high-risk situations and the use of water as a strategy is not usually recommended. In this situation the midwife will need to carefully read Verity's notes as this plan may have been arranged during pregnancy.

Further questions specific to Scenario 1 include:

1. Do other members of the team already know about this situation?
2. Who should the midwife inform about this request?
3. Is there any evidence to show that this request is unsafe for Verity or her baby?
4. How can the midwife support Verity in her request?
5. How does the midwife prepare the environment appropriately?
6. Where should Amanda document information?

Scenario 2

Chloe is now 36 weeks pregnant with her first baby and reveals to Samantha, her midwife, that she is very scared about labour as she was abused as a child.

Practice point

Women who are survivors of abusive situations require special care when in labour. Often they do not reveal this information in the antenatal period but in this scenario Samantha has time to make some preparations in order to provide the best care for Chloe.

Further questions specific to Scenario 2 include:

1. What is the best model of care that could be used to care for Chloe?
2. Who is the best person to care for her in labour?
3. Who else should Samantha discuss this situation with, with Chloe's permission?
4. In labour what strategies would be the best to help Chloe?
5. Which ones are not likely to be the most helpful?
6. How will the midwife ensure Chloe is central to her care?

Conclusion

There are many remedies and strategies that women may choose to employ when faced with the hard work of labour. The midwife must respect the woman's unique circumstances and her individual tolerance of pain when discussing the options available to her. However, the midwife must acknowledge the limits of her own professional competence and seek the support and guidance of her colleagues when a woman's request falls outside her sphere of practice. The midwife has an important role in enhancing the woman's confidence in her ability to cope with her pain but must also recognize the place for pharmacological methods when needed or requested by the woman.

Resources

British Acupuncture Council: Pain relief during labour. http://www.gloucesteracupuncture. co.uk/painreliefdurringlabour. htm.

Hypnobirthing: http://www. thehypnobirthingcentre.co.uk/ ?gclid=CJK44Ozb6pQCFRuD1Qod PQ96Rg.

National Childbirth Trust: Active birth. http://www.nctpregnancyandbabycare. com/info-centre/a-to-z/view/3.

Patient UK: Pain relief in labour. http://www.patient.co.uk/ showdoc/40000218/.

Women's health Matters: Massage. http:// www.womenshealthmatters.ca/Centres/ pregnancy/childbirth/massage.html.

References

Allahbadia G, Vaidya P: Why deliver in the supine position? *Australian and New Zealand Journal of Obstetrics and Gynaecology* 32:104–106, 1992.

Allaire A, Moos M, Wells S: Complementary and alternative medicine in pregnancy: a survey of North Carolina certified nurse-midwives, *Obstetrics & Gynecology* 95(1):19–23, 2000.

Anderson T: Time to throw the waterbirth thermometer away? *MIDIRS Midwifery Digest* 14(3):370–374, 2004.

Bowler E: Just a normal disabled Mum, *The Practising Midwife* 11(7):1 5–16, 2008.

Brown J, Brown A: Improving provision in a maternity unit: a case study, *The Practising Midwife* 6(7):21, 2003.

Buckley S: Ecstatic birth: nature's hormonal blueprint for labor, 2005. Online. Available http://www. sarahjbuckley.com/articles/ecstatic-birth.htm. September 30, 2008.

Carroll D, Tramer M, McQuay H, et al: Transcutaneous electrical nerve stimulation in labour pain: a systematic review, *British Journal of Obsterics and Gynaecology* 104(2):169–175, 1997.

Chang M, Wang S, Chen C: Issues and innovations in nursing practice. Effects of massage on pain and anxiety during labour: a randomized controlled trial in Taiwan, *Journal of Advanced Nursing* 38(1):68–73, 2002.

Cluett ER, Nikodem VC, McCandlish RE, et al: Immersion in water in pregnancy, labour and birth DOI: 10.1002/14651858.CD000111.pub2, *Cochrane Database of Systematic Reviews* 1(CD000111), 2002.

Coates T: Transcutaneous electrical nerve stimulation: TENS, *The Practising Midwife* 1(11):12–14, 1998.

Davis P: *Aromatherapy, An A-Z*, Saffron Walden, 1991, CW Daniel.

de Jong P, Johanson R, Baxen P, et al: Randomised trial comparing the upright and supine positions for the second stage of labour, *British Journal of Obsterics and Gynaecology* 106(3): 291–292, 1999.

Dhany A: Essential oils and massage in intrapartum care, *The Practising Midwife* 11(5):34–39, 2008.

Eberhard J, Stein S, Geissbuehler V: Experience of pain and analgesia with water and land births, *Journal of Psychosomatic Obstetrics & Gynecology* 26(2):127–133, 2005. http://www. informaworld.com/smpp/title-content =t713634100-db=jour-tab=issueslist -branches=26-v26.

Eriksson M, Ladfors L, Mattsson L, et al: Warm tub bath during labour: a study of 1385 women with pre-labour rupture of the membranes after 34 weeks of gestation, *Acta Obstetrica et Gynecologica Scandinavica* 75:642–644, 1996.

Field T, Hermandez-Reif M, Taylor S, et al: Labour pain is reduced by massage therapy, *Journal of Psychosomatic Obstetrics and Gynaecology* 18: 286–291, 1997.

Green J: Expectations and experiences of pain in labour: findings from a large prospective study, *Birth* 20(2): 65–72, 1993.

Green J, Coupland V, Kitzinger J: *Great expectations. A prospective study of women's expectations and experiences of childbirth*, Hale, 1998, Books for Midwives Press.

Hall J: *Midwifery mind and spirit: emerging issues of care*, Oxford, 2001, Books for Midwives.

Hall J, Taylor M: Birth and spirituality. In Downe S, editor: *Normal childbirth: evidence and debate*, Edinburgh, 2008, Churchill Livingstone.

Hall SM, Holloway IM: Staying in control: women's experiences of labour in water, *Midwifery* 14:30–36, 1998.

Hamilton A: Pain relief and comfort in labour. In Fraser DM, Cooper MA, editors: *Myles textbook for midwives*, ed 14, Edinburgh, 2003, Churchill Livingstone.

Hodnett ED: Pain and women's satisfaction with the experience of childbirth: a systematic review, *American Journal of Obstetrics and Gynecology (supplement)* 186(5):S160–S172, 2002.

Hodnett ED, Gates S, Hofmeyr GJ, et al: Continuous support for women during childbirth, *Cochrane Database of Systematic Reviews* 2(CD003766), 2007, DOI: 10.1002/14651858.CD003766.pub2.

Kimber L: Massage for childbirth and pregnancy, *The Practising Midwife* 5(3):20–23, 2002.

Kimber L, McNabb M, Mc Court C, et al: Massage or music for pain relief in labour: a pilot randomised placebo controlled trial Online. Available doi:10.1016/j.ejpain 4 Jan 2008, *European Journal of Pain*, 2008.

Kitzinger S: Authoritative touch in childbirth: a cross-cultural approach. In Davis-Floyd RE, Sargent CF, editors: *Childbirth and authoritative knowledge: cross-cultural perspectives*, Berkeley, 1997, University of California Press.

Lally JE, Murtagh MJ, Macphail S, et al: More in hope than expectation: a systematic review of women's expectations and experience of pain relief in labour, *BMC Medicine* 6(7):1–10, 2008. Online. Available http://www.biomedcentral.com/1741-7015/6/7/ abstract 5 Dec 2008.

Leap N, Anderson T: The role of pain in normal birth and the empowerment of women. In Downe S, editor: *Normal childbirth: evidence and debate*, Edinburgh, 2008, Churchill Livingstone.

Lowe NK: Explaining the pain of active labour: the importance of maternal confidence, *Research in Nursing and Health* 12:237–245, 1989.

Mitchell M, Doyle M: Complementary therapies in the midwifery curriculum 2: development and evaluation of a CT module, *The Practising Midwife* 5(4):39, 2002.

Mitchell M, Williams J, Hobbs E, et al, *British Journal of Midwifery* 14(10):576–582, 2006.

National Institute for Health and Clinical Excellence (NICE): *Intrapartum care. *Care of healthy women and their babies during childbirth*. NICE clinical guideline 55, London, 2007, NICE.

Niven C, Gijspers K: Obstetric and non-obstetric factors related to labour pain, *Journal of Reproductive and Infant Psychology* 2:61–78, 1990.

Niven C, Murphy-Black T: Memory for labor pain: a review of the literature, *Birth* 22(4):244–253, 2000.

Nursing and Midwifery Council (NMC): *Midwives rules and code of practice*, London, 2004, NMC.

Nursing and Midwifery Council (NMC): *Standards for medicines management*, London, 2007a, NMC.

Nursing and Midwifery Council (NMC): *Record keeping advice sheet*. Online. Available http://www.nmc-uk.org/ aFrameDisplay.aspx?DocumentID=4008 July 1 08, London, 2007b, NMC.

Odent M: *The farmer and the obstetrician*, London, 2002, Free Association Books.

Ramnero A, Hanson U, Kihlgren M: Acupuncture treatment during labour – a randomised controlled trial, *Bjog-an International Journal of Obstetrics and Gynaecology* 109:637–644, 2002.

Saisto T: Obstetric, psychosocial and pain-related background, and treatment of fear of childbirth. Unpublished dissertation. University of Helsinki, Institute of Clinical Medicine, Department of Obstetrics and Gynecology, Faculty of Medicine, 2001. Online. Available https://oa.doria.fi/ bitstream/handle/10024/2281/obstetri. pdf?sequence=1. July 30, 2008.

Seymour J: Pain relief in childbirth, *Nursing Times* 93(20):55–56, 1997.

Simkin PP, O'Hara M: Nonpharmacologic relief of pain during labour: systematic reviews of five methods, *American Journal of Obstetrics and Gynecology (supplement)* 186(5):S131–S159, 2002.

Smith CA, Collins CT, Cyna AM, et al: Complementary and alternative therapies for pain management in labour, *Cochrane Database of Systematic Reviews* 2(CD003521), 2006, DOI: 10.1002/14651858. CD003521.pub2.

Spiby H, Slade P, Escott D, et al: Selected coping strategies in labour: an investigation of women's experiences, *Birth* 30(3):189–194, 2003.

Thompson F: *Mothers and midwives: the ethical journey*, Oxford, 2004, Books for Midwives.

Tiran D: Complementary therapies: time to regulate?, *The Practising Midwife* 10(3):14–19, 2007.

Tritten J: Traditional midwives. Roots of complementary therapies?, *The Practising Midwife* 5(4):17, 2002.

van der Ploeg J, Vervest H, Liem A, et al: Transcutaneous nerve stimulation (TENS) during the first stage of labour: a randomised clinical trial, *Pain* 68:75–78, 1996.

Waldenstrom U: Women's memory of childbirth at two months and one year after the birth, *Birth* 30(4): 248–254, 2003.

Waldenstrom U, Bergman V, Vasell G: The complexity of labor pain: experiences of 278 women, *Journal of Psychosomatic Obstetrics and Gynaecology* 17:215–228, 1996.

Walsh D: *Evidence-based care of normal labour and birth*, London, 2007, Routledge.

Chapter 5

Using water in labour

Trigger scenario

Emma responds to a call from Yasmin's partner to say that she is now in labour and would like the midwife to come to their home. On arrival at the house Emma finds Yasmin resting in a birthing pool in their sitting room, which they have rented for the occasion.

Introduction

The use of water in labour has become more acceptable in recent years. In Europe, the use of water was advocated as a source of relaxation (Odent 1984), in response to the pioneering work of Igor Tjarkovsky in Russia (Mackey 2001). However, it is believed that in other countries, water has been a source of comfort for labouring women throughout history (Garland 2006a). There are links with the use of water in labour and the spiritual nature of birth (Garland 2000, Wickham 2001). The increased desire of women to choose to labour in water worldwide has subsequently led to an increase of birth in water, websites relating to the subject and companies providing pools, both to women direct at home and to birthing units.

There is evidence to show that the use of water in the first stage of labour has benefits, including higher feelings of control by women (Hall & Holloway 1998) experiencing less pain (Cluett et al 2002, Eberhard et al 2005), less use of augmentation by Syntocinon and less need for epidurals (Cluett et al 2004, Eberhard et al 2005). The aim of this chapter is to consider the issues surrounding the use of water in labour and birth, both at home and in an institutional setting, and the role of the midwife in these situations. This chapter should be read alongside Chapter 4 relating to 'Non-pharmacological methods of coping with labour'.

Antenatal preparation

As the use of a warm pool or bath in labour is becoming increasingly common, midwives should be active in discussing this option with women in the antenatal period. The midwife needs to be aware of local policies relating to labour and birth in water and able to give the appropriate information to women about the resources available. The woman should be encouraged to consider the advantages and disadvantages of using water for both labour and birth. Explanation regarding policy about the birth of the third stage should also be given. If a woman is wishing for a home water birth the midwife should ensure she is confident in the care of women in the situation. If she is not confident she should approach her supervisor of midwives to put a plan of action in place to develop her skills and knowledge in this area. She may be able to access local study days or in-service education and spend time working with another midwife who is already proficient in the use of water for labour and birth.

The midwife will also need to be aware of sources where women may purchase or rent pools for home use, as well as what is available in the local maternity units. Knowledge of the accessibility and availability of pools should lead to the appropriate choice for the individual woman of the place of birth. Midwives can also help women prepare the home for the birth and ensure there is sufficient room for the pool, safety in the home and provision of equipment. A 'practice run' for the birth should take place

to ensure the equipment is working effectively and that it is situated in an appropriate place. In some situations it may be necessary to obtain a structural survey for a property should a pool be situated upstairs as water is very heavy. Assessment of the length of time to fill the pool should be made as well as consideration of how a woman will get out of the pool in an emergency.

Activity

Find out which local units have birth pools. How often are they in use?

How frequently are women turned away from using it due to it being in use?

Access the Home birth website and find out about the different pools available to women at home: http://www.homebirth.org.uk/water.htm

Labour in water

The use of a warm water bath during labour is a valuable way to relieve pain (Cluett et al 2002, Eberhard et al 2005). The *NICE intrapartum care guideline* advocates that women should have the opportunity to use water for pain relief during labour (NICE 2007:19). The use of a bath or shower may also be of benefit, particularly during early labour. However, the depth of the pool to the level of a woman's breast is thought to be more appropriate and women appear to welcome a large enough pool to enable the ability to move around (Maude & Foureur 2007).

It is stated that any woman who has an uncomplicated pregnancy and is experiencing a straightforward labour should be recommended to use water in labour (RCOG/RCM 2006, NICE 2007). However there are suggestions that women who have hypertension may also benefit from the relaxing properties of water in pregnancy (Katz 2003), though this is yet to be investigated in labour. There are also reports of twins and babies presenting by the breech being born in water (Evans 1997). Appropriately assessed women who have had a previous caesarean section have successfully used water in labour (Garland 2006b), however local midwifery guidelines often limit the use of a birthing pool to women with an uncomplicated obstetric history. Further research regarding the use of water in labour is urgently needed to enable women with a range of obstetric backgrounds, to use a pool with confidence.

Activity

Find out in your area which women are recommended to use water in labour.
What evidence are these criteria are based on?
Find out what your local labour guidelines say about when a woman should get into the pool.
What evidence are these criteria based on?

Practical issues

According to NICE (2007) there is insufficient evidence to suggest when the best time is for a woman to get into a birth pool. Michel Odent (1997) suggests there is benefit for women to wait to enter the pool until labour has become established. It is suggested that the anticipation of getting in the water, including listening to the water fill and seeing it, may help women lose their inhibitions and also be significant in the process of the labour (Odent 1997, Maude & Foureur 2007).

In the hospital situation the midwife will need to prepare the pool for use. She will need to establish if it is clean, if all equipment is ready and will need to fill the pool. Box 5.1 explains the equipment that should be available for a pool birth.

Activity

Find out:

- how long it takes to fill the pool in your local unit
- how the birthing pool is cleaned between births, who carries this out and how long it should 'rest' between births.

Tricia Anderson (2004) examined the evidence around the optimum temperature of the water and maintained that women in labour in a birth pool should be able to decide for themselves if it is too hot or cold (also see Geissbuehler et al 2002). However, anxieties over potential risks of hyperthermia to mother and baby led NICE (2007:19) to advise that the temperature of the water should be maintained below 37.5°C. This means that monitoring should take place of the water temperature. The woman's partner can help by adding hot or cold water as the woman requires.

Box 5.1 Equipment required

- **A deep pool**
Rationale So that the woman may deeply immerse and move around

- **Step, or access to pool**
Rationale For woman to get in and out easily; for midwife to access if required

- **Equipment to fill and empty it with hot and cold water**
Rationale To maintain a comfortable temperature for the woman

- **Thermometer for pool**
Rationale To check temperature of water hourly

- **Thermometer for mum**
Rationale To ensure she is not hypo-or hyperthermic

- **Plenty of towels**
Rationale For when the woman wishes to get out of the water

- **Waterproof floor and furniture protector if in the home**
Rationale To protect the floor and furniture from splashes

- **Mirror (some midwives use a tile)**
Rationale To visualize the emerging baby on the bottom of the pool

- **Torch and spare batteries**
Rationale To visualize the baby in dim lighting

- **Sieve**
Rationale For removing debris from the pool

- **Something for the midwife to kneel or sit on**
Rationale For the comfort of the midwife

- **A waterproof Doppler or pinard**
Rationale To monitor the fetal heart rate

- **Long gloves if required**
Rationale To protect the midwife's arms

- **Complete change of clothes for midwife**
Rationale In case the midwife gets wet

- **Something for the woman to lie down on (mattress, sofa, bed)**
Rationale In case she wishes to get out of the water and rest and for after the birth

- **A birth stool (hospital)**
Rationale For the woman to sit on for the third stage

- **A bucket or dish**
Rationale To 'catch' the placenta and membranes in

- **Resuscitation equipment**
Rationale To resuscitate the baby if required in emergency

Activity

Find out what type of thermometer is used for water births in your unit.
Find out how the thermometer is sterilized between births.

First stage of labour care

Monitoring should also take place of the woman's temperature on an hourly basis (NICE 2007:19) and monitoring of the fetal heart in accordance with the usual labour guidelines (NICE 2007).

A midwife should consider how she is going to carry this out. She may need to consider whether she needs something to stand on to reach into the water, if the woman will be expected to stand up and whether there is electronic equipment suitable for underwater use. She will also need to think about what clothing she will need to wear for the labour as she could become wet. An extra set of clothes is advisable, and she may require elbow length gloves. Vaginal examinations, if required, may be carried out in the water, or the woman may prefer to get out for this. Record keeping should be exemplary in accordance with the rules of practice (NMC 2004).

Women may choose to use only the pool as a form of pain relief and successfully give birth in the water. However, some women may also use other methods. If a woman has been using a TENS machine she will need to remove this prior to getting into the water.

Women may use Entonox while they are in the water, but it is important that they are not left alone with this, in case it causes drowsiness. In the *NICE intrapartum guidelines* (2007:21) it states:

Women should not enter water (a birthing pool or bath) within 2 hours of opioid administration or if they feel drowsy.

During the first stage of labour the partner should be encouraged to be close to the woman and to provide comfort if she wishes. In some situations the partner may also wish to be in the water. Their choice should be respected, though the partner should be requested to wear a costume of some kind when the midwife is present.

Second stage of labour care

In situations where women wish to remain in the water for the birth midwives should maintain a 'hands-off' approach as much as possible to prevent unnecessary stimulation of the baby. Usually a second midwife will be present to provide support if needed. There have been suggestions that more perineal trauma may occur in water births. However, studies are showing that women appear to have more intact perineums (Geissbuehler et al 2004), less rectal sphincter damage and less perineal trauma overall (Otigbah et al 2000). A mirror and torch may be used to observe the emerging baby. The baby should be born completely under water and then brought to the surface gently in case the baby has a short umbilical cord.

Activity

Find out who is regarded as 'experienced' about water birth in your area and talk to them about what their experience has taught them.

Third stage of labour care

As the first and second stages of a water birth are likely to have been physiological in nature it is probable that the third stage may be birthed physiologically as well. If the woman desires, this may take place in the pool, though caution about assessment of blood loss should be noted. In water, blood will be dispersed and the woman may feel uncomfortable in seeing or sitting in this. Careful observation of her clinical condition while she is still in the water should be made, in case of unrecognized haemorrhage. In other situations the pool may be drained for the third stage or the woman may be helped out of the pool to deliver the third stage according to usual land birth practices.

Activity

Find out the policy for third stage care in your local area.

What evidence are these policies based on?

Care of the baby after water birth

As with birth in any situation the care of the baby involves vigilance to observe behaviour to ensure respiration is initially established and maintained. Tricia Anderson (2004) notes that babies born in water may take a bit longer to establish respiration and their skin remains blue in colour for longer. The reasons for this potential delay may be multfactorial (Garland 2000). If the baby does not need resuscitation he may lie in the water with his body in the water and the face above held by the woman in order to retain his body heat. The issue of potential hypothermia after birth is of concern, therefore maintaining the appropriate temperature of the water, ensuring skin-to-skin contact and observation of the breathing patterns of the baby are important. Once the woman

leaves the water the baby's temperature should be checked and care provided as per normal, such as skin-to-skin contact and breastfeeding if the woman wishes.

Emergency issues

As in any birth, midwives must be vigilant for any deviations from normal. In any situations of concern the woman should be encouraged to get out of the water in order for further assessment to take place and, in a fixed pool, the water may be drained. In the 'practice run' mentioned previously it is advisable to consider with the woman and her partner how the woman would get out in an emergency. Water embolism has been suggested as a potential problem in water births. However, this is a hypothetical risk (Wickham 2005), but midwives should be prepared with regard to how to deal with a collapsed woman in a pool. Potential emergencies, such as haemorrhage and shoulder dystocia may also occur (but rarely) and consideration should be made of these possibilities. In cases where babies require resuscitation a flat space next to the pool should be available in the home, and resuscitation equipment accessible in the hospital.

Activity

Find out if there is any training about emergencies in water births in your area.

What happens at water birth emergencies?

Make sure you know how the pool should be cleaned after use.

Reflection on trigger

Look back on the trigger scenario at the start of the chapter.

Emma responds to a call from Yasmin's partner to say that she is now in labour and would like the midwife to come to their home. On arrival at the house Emma finds Yasmin resting in a birthing pool in their sitting room, which they have rented for the occasion.

The scenario is one that a community-based midwife could face if she is called to a woman labouring at home. It is possible the midwife is aware that the couple have chosen to use a birthing pool, and it is possible this may not have been communicated to her. This raises issues of communication as well as choice and safety. Now that you are familiar with the use of water in labour you should have insight into how the scenario relates to the evidence. The jigsaw model will now be used to explore the trigger scenario in more depth.

Effective communication

As in all areas of midwifery practice, communication with regard to the use of water in labour is important. During the antenatal period midwives should ask about women's plans for relaxation and relief during labour as well as providing appropriate information on availability of resources for women. Questions that arise from the scenario might include: Had Emma met Yasmin before? Did she know that Yasmin is planning a birthing pool? Has this been discussed in the antenatal period? Does Emma need to

document Yasmin's use of a pool and where will this be written? Who else might Emma need to communicate with in relation to Yasmin's choice?

Woman-centred care

This involves giving women choice that also includes the evidence that is available. NICE (2007:33) advise that: 'women should be informed that there is insufficient high-quality evidence to either support or discourage giving birth in water.' This places the onus on the woman to make her choice about her use of water and for a midwife to support her in this choice. Availability of pools in birth units may be a factor in women's desires to choose that centre or to rent one for use at home. Questions that arise from the scenario might include: Has Yasmin been given all the evidence surrounding the use of water in labour and by whom? Has she been facilitated in this choice by Emma or has she made this choice with her partner alone? How can the use of water in labour help women feel central to their care?

Using best evidence

As indicated in the above section, according to NICE there is currently insufficient research evidence to show whether the use of water is of benefit or otherwise. However, there is some evidence showing that women require less analgesia and there is an increase in satisfaction (Cluett et al 2002). However, there is increasing evidence of women's and midwives stories about their experiences of labour and birth in water (e.g. Maude & Foureur 2007). Questions that arise from the scenario might include: What is the evidence regarding appropriate care of women in a pool in labour? What is the evidence regarding the birth of the baby under water? What is the evidence around the birth of the placenta in water? Is there guidance from NICE around care in labour in water (NICE 2007)?

Professional and legal issues

The current low frequency of water births that takes place means that some midwives may never come across a woman who wishes for one. It is therefore important that midwives should keep up-to-date with advances in water birth research and that training needs are met to ensure they are prepared for women who choose this option (RCOG/RCM 2006). Questions that arise from the scenario might include: Is Emma sufficiently trained and competent to support Yasmin if she chooses to give birth in water? If Emma does not feel experienced or competent, whom should she make contact with? How should Emma's competence be assessed and her confidence increased? What should Emma do if Yasmin does not fulfil the local criteria for a pool birth?

Team working

In a home situation a midwife will often be working in tandem with another colleague or within a team. This means that she would often call a second midwife to provide support for the latter stages of labour. A midwife may also

need to be working with those who are providing support for the woman: her partner, family members or a doula who has been employed to provide support in situations where there is poor continuity. A supervisor of midwives will also be accessible to support the midwife. The midwife also works within a primary care team or in a hospital setting, alongside other midwives and a medical team. Questions that arise from the scenario might include: Does Emma need to contact another midwife; if so when will this be? Do Yasmin and her partner have other members of the family or another support person in the home? Does Emma need to contact her supervisor for any reason? Do all members of the multi-professional team support the use of water for labour and birth? Who was involved in the development of the local pool birth policy?

Clinical dexterity

Care for a woman in the pool requires the same dexterity as the care of any woman in labour. In fact there is potential that use of pools in labour will mean midwives 'interfere' less in labour. Monitoring the wellbeing of the baby may require some dexterity and negotiation with the woman to move if required. Questions that arise from the scenario might include: Has Emma participated in a water birth before? Is the pool in an appropriate area to make manoeuvring easy?

Models of care

Labour in water may take place both in home and hospital settings as indicated.

In the community setting a midwife may be working as part of a team or with a colleague. All midwives work in multi-disciplinary teams. Questions that arise from the scenario might include: Does Emma have a colleague who is available for support if required? If so, how can she access them? When should she make contact with this person? In an emergency whom will she call? Is there local provision for one-to-one care in labour?

Safe environment

Generally, labouring in water is considered safe for the low-risk woman and her baby. There have been situations where a baby has been born compromised (Gilbert & Tookey 1999), as in any situation. The midwife should ensure the pool is situated in a safe place in the home, away from electric cables, plugs and equipment that could be splashed. In addition, health and safety concerns about the wellbeing of the midwife should be considered, especially in relation to straining her back or knees. Questions that arise from the scenario might include: Is the pool situated safely? Is the structure of the building safe? Can Emma give care to Yasmin without harming herself? How will Yasmin move out of the pool in an emergency? What special equipment is required to enhance the safety of the midwife, the woman and her baby?

Promotes health

The current available evidence shows that a woman using the pool for labour may require less pain relief from pharmacological methods, and less augmentation with Syntocinon (Cluett et al 2002). Therefore this would indicate water in labour will promote the wellbeing of both mother and baby. Questions that arise from the scenario might include: Are there medical reasons why a woman may not use a pool? Is there any evidence that pool birth promotes the initiation or continuation of breastfeeding? How might pool birth enhance a woman's sense of wellbeing? How might the use of water in labour encourage the partner to be more involved in the birthing process?

Further scenarios

The following scenarios enable you to consider how specific situations influence the care the midwife provides. Use the jigsaw model to explore the issues raised in the scenario.

Scenario 1

Melanie is caring for Simone as she labours in a pool with her second baby in the hospital birth unit. When she climbed in her cervix had dilated to 5 cm. Melanie notes that the water has become discoloured by what looks like fresh meconium.

Practice point

Serious consideration should be given to the presence of meconium in the liquor as a potential indication of fetal compromise. However, in water meconium may also not be an indication of compromise but of other things (see http://www.homebirth.org.uk/meconium.htm#2). Careful assessment needs to be made of the situation.

Further questions specific to Scenario 1 include:

1. What are the potential causes for the meconium being present?
2. What should Melanie communicate to Simone?
3. Should she ask Simone to get out of the pool?
4. What observations should be carried out?
5. Whom should she inform on the unit about the meconium?
6. Where should the information be documented?

Scenario 2

Danielle has arrived for her booking appointment. Lynn, her midwife, notes that Danielle walks with crutches and subsequently discovers that she has a form of cerebral palsy. Danielle indicates that she would like to labour in the pool at the unit and asks if this would be a problem.

Practice point

In situations where women have disability, discussion regarding care in labour should take place early, and be ongoing, in order to plan the best form of care for her. This will include other members of the multi-disciplinary team to ensure a full assessment may

be made. In relation to labour in water particular attention should be made to the woman's physical ability to get in and out of the pool. If required, lifting equipment should be made available.

Further questions specific to Scenario 2 include:

1. How can Lynn ensure Danielle is central to her care?
2. Who will also provide support to Danielle throughout pregnancy and birth?
3. Who will need to be informed about Danielle's request?
4. How will Lynn present the options available to Danielle?
5. What will Lynn document and where?

Conclusion

The use of water in labour is to be encouraged for women experiencing a straightforward pregnancy and labour. Midwives should therefore become familiar with the issues around the use of water and pool accessibility in the local area. The community midwife has a particular role to play in supporting women access the information they require to make informed choice about this option and to help enable them select the appropriate place for birth. Midwives should be up-to-date in current evidence, trained and prepared to facilitate birth in water at home or in the maternity unit as required.

Useful resources

Sheila Kitzinger's water birth pages: http://www.sheilakitzinger.com/ WaterBirth.htm.

Waterbirth International: http://www.waterbirth.org/mc/ page.do.

Waterbirth website: http://www. waterbirthinfo.com/.

Waterbirth pages: http://www. homebirth.org.uk/.

Photographs of water birth: *The Practising Midwife*. June 2008.

References

Anderson T: Time to throw the waterbirth thermometer away? *MIDIRS Midwifery Digest* 14(3):370–374, 2004.

Cluett ER, Nikodem VC, McCandlish RE, et al: Immersion in water in pregnancy, labour and birth DOI: 10.1002/14651858.CD000111. pub2, Cochrane Database of Systematic Reviews 1(CD000111), 2002.

Cluett ER, Pickering RM, Getliffe K, et al: Randomised controlled trial of labouring in water compared with standard of augmentation for management of dystocia in first stage of labour, *BMJ* 328(7435):314, 2004.

Eberhard J, Stein S, Geissbuehler V: Experience of pain and analgesia with water and land births, *Journal of Psychosomatic Obstetrics & Gynecology* 26(2):127–133, 2005.

Evans J: Can a twin birth be a positive experience? *Midwifery Matters* 74:6–11, 1997.

Garland D: *Waterbirth: an attitude to care*, Oxford, 2000, Books for Midwives.

Garland D: Waterbirth – an international overview: Dianne Garland, a freelance UK-based midwife lecturer, spoke at the ICM Brisbane Congress and now gives an update on the practice of waterbirth around the world. International Midwifery, 2006a. Online. Available http://findarticles.com/p/articles/ mi_m0KTL/is_2_19/ai_n17213917/pg_ 1?tag=artBody;col1. June 22, 2008.

Garland D: Is waterbirth a 'safe and realistic' option for women following a previous caesarean section? Completion of a three year data study, *MIDIRS Midwifery Digest* 16(2):217–220, 2006b.

Geissbuehler V, Eberhard J, Lebrecht A: Waterbirth: water temperature and bathing time – mother knows best! *Journal of Perinatal Medicine* 30:371–378, 2002.

Geissbuehler V, Stein S, Eberhard J: Waterbirth compared with land births: an observational study of nine years, *Journal of Perinatal Medicine* 32(4):308–314, 2004.

Gilbert RE, Tookey PA: Perinatal mortality and morbidity among babies delivered in water: surveillance study and postal survey, *British Medical Journal* 319(7208):483–487, 1999.

Hall S, Holloway I: Staying in control: women's experiences of labour in water, *Midwifery* 14(1):30–36, 1998.

Katz VL: Exercise in water during pregnancy, *Clinical Obstetrics and Gynecology* 46(2):432–441, 2003.

Mackey MM: Use of water in labor and birth, *Clinical Obstetrics & Gynecology* 44(4):733–749, 2001.

Maude RM, Foureur MJ: It's beyond water: stories of women's experience of using water for labour and birth, *Women and Birth* 20:17–24, 2007.

National Institute for Health and Clinical Excellence (NICE): *Intrapartum care of healthy women and their babies during childbirth*, London, 2007, RCOG Press.

Nursing and Midwifery Council (NMC): *Midwives rules and standards*, London, 2004, NMC.

Odent M: *Birth reborn: what birth can and should be*, London, 1984, Fontana.

Odent M: Can water immersion stop labor? *Journal of Nurse-Midwifery* 42(5):414–416, 1997.

Otigbah C, Dhanjal MK, Harmsworth G, et al: A retrospective comparison of water births and conventional vaginal deliveries, *European Journal of Obstetrics & Gynecology and Reproductive Biology* 91(1):15–20, 2000.

RCOG/Royal College of Midwives: Joint statement No 1. Immersion in water during labour and birth, 2006. Online. Available http://www.rcog.org.uk/index.asp?PageID=546. July 30, 2008.

Wickham S: Reclaiming spirituality in birth, 2001. Online. Available http://www.withwoman.co.uk/contents/info/spiritualbirth.html. October 20, 2007.

Wickham S: The birth of water embolism, *The Practising Midwife* 8(11):37, 2005.

Chapter 6

Pharmacological methods of pain relief

Trigger scenario

Siân is in active labour with her first baby. She has been using breathing and relaxation techniques but during her last contraction she asked for an epidural. Her partner looks shocked. Siân's birth plan states quite clearly that she does not plan to have one.

Introduction

Although women no longer need to experience the pain associated with childbirth, the decision regarding whether or not to use pharmacological methods of analgesia is not straightforward. Women vary in their hopes and fears regarding the childbirth experience. Some want to cope with as little pain relief as possible and others want a pain-free birth. The increasing use of technology throughout maternity care, including induction,

acceleration and electronic monitoring of labour, has increased the need for effective means of alleviating the associated pain.

Despite the wide availability of epidural services, however, an increasing proportion of women are very worried about the thought of pain in labour. A prospective study exploring women's expectations and experiences of intrapartum care in 2000 and comparing them with data from women in 1987 found that 26% of primigravidae in 2000 reported feeling 'very worried' about the thought of pain in labour compared with 9% in 1987 (Green et al 2003).

Much emphasis is placed in current maternity provision on the maxim that women should be fully informed and involved in decisions about their care (Department of Health 2007a, 2007b, Maternity Care Working Party 2007, NICE 2007). Although ideally women should receive information and consider the options before they are distracted by painful uterine contractions, they will inevitably face decisions about their care during labour. To participate actively, the woman needs to remain awake and fully aware of what is happening around her but at the same time, she needs to be able to cope with her pain. Thus, finding analgesia that does not oversedate but is relatively effective is a particular challenge for the woman who requests pharmacological means of pain relief.

This chapter focuses on inhalational, opioid and epidural analgesia.

(See Chapters 4 and 5 for non-pharmacological methods.)

Inhalational analgesia

When pain relief is achieved by breathing in an anaesthetic gas, this is referred to as inhalational analgesia. The fact that the overall concentration of the gas is much less than would be administered if an anaesthetic were required means that the woman remains conscious. However, the fact that it is an anaesthetic agent should alert the midwife to the importance of maintaining careful observation of the woman's wellbeing.

Nitrous oxide is the only form of inhalational analgesia available in the UK. It is provided for women in labour as a mixture of 50% nitrous oxide and 50% oxygen and is commonly known as Entonox. It is valuable as it can be used while other forms of analgesia are being prepared or taking effect.

Method of administration

Self-administration prevents overdose and anaesthesia being induced. For this reason it is important that the midwife informs the birth partner not to help the woman by holding the mask over her face.

Some coordination is required to achieve optimum benefit from Entonox. As it takes 20–60 seconds to take effect, the woman needs to start using it as soon as a contraction begins, rather than when it has reached its peak. The student midwife can help by placing a hand on the fundus and detecting the contraction before it becomes painful to the woman. Thus the student can inform the woman when to start using the Entonox and to stop when the peak of the contraction has been overcome.

It must be explained to the woman that the gas is not being released constantly from the mask but that it requires the woman to take sufficiently deep breaths in order to open the valve. The woman needs to press the mask firmly over her nose and mouth to form a tight seal. She should then be encouraged to take deep, slow breaths, keeping the mask on her face for both inspiration and expiration. The Entonox apparatus makes a characteristically deeper noise when the valve opens, following the correct breathing technique.

It is important that the woman removes the mask from her face in between contractions to enable her to breathe some fresh air and regain her awareness. Entonox is quickly excreted via the lungs and she should feel her usual self within about 2 minutes.

Some women do not like the thought of breathing into a mask. They may associate the sensation with going to the dentist and might prefer to use a mouthpiece. The woman will require frequent sips of water; this method causes the mouth to feel very dry as water is lost in expired air.

Activity

Make sure you know which of the midwives rules provide guidance in relation to the equipment used for administering inhalational analgesics.

Find out what temperature Entonox should be stored at.

Impact on the woman

The longstanding and continued use of Entonox in labour reflects its relative safety as a pharmacological method of analgesia. However, inappropriate use of Entonox can lead to hyperventilation and associated hypoxia, dizziness and tetany (Jordan 2002). Therefore, a woman using Entonox must have her respiration rate closely observed and complaints of tingling or spasm in her hands or feet should lead to

suspension of its use. In a study comparing the effects of Entonox and epidural analgesia on arterial oxygen saturation in labour (Arfeen et al 1994) it was reported that women who used Entonox had longer and more severe hypoxic episodes than women who had an epidural.

In addition, women using Entonox may suddenly feel nauseous and light-headed (NICE 2007). The midwife supporting her must be prepared for this (vomit bowl and tissues to hand) and ensure that she is positioned to avoid aspiration. A cool facecloth placed on the back of the woman's neck or forehead may alleviate such symptoms in between use.

Prolonged occupational exposure to Entonox has been associated with spontaneous abortion and congenital abnormality (BOC 1999).

Activity

Find out what measures are taken where you work to reduce employees' exposure to waste anaesthetic gases.

Investigate what regulations govern the safe use of Entonox in the workplace.

Impact on the baby

Entonox is excreted via the lungs of the neonate, usually within 2 to 3 minutes of the birth. Respiratory depression associated with the combined use of opioids and Entonox may delay this process.

Opioid analgesia

What are opioids?

An opioid drug is one that attaches itself to the body's opioid receptors – that is, those that respond to endorphins and enkephalins (Jordan 2002). Opioids used in midwifery practice include pethidine, diamorphine and meptazinol. They are 'controlled drugs' which means that their use is closely monitored under legislation by the Misuse of Drugs Act 1971 and they fall into Class A. These classes are used to enable penalties to be attributed to their abuse. Controlled drugs are further categorized according to the Misuse of Drugs Regulations 2001, which provides guidance on how they should be stored and administered: opioids fall under Schedule 2. The Health Act (2006) introduced comprehensive governance arrangements for the monitoring and inspection of controlled drugs. It also introduced standard operating procedures (SOPs) for the use and management of controlled drugs and the requirement that all healthcare organizations should have an Accountable Officer to oversee these arrangements. In addition to the legislation on the administration of controlled drugs and professional guidance (NMC 2007), individual NHS trusts have their own frameworks for safe practice (Department of Health 2007c). NICE (2007) recommend that opioids should be available for women to use in all birth settings.

Route of administration

Opioids are usually given by intramuscular injection during labour. It is common practice for intramuscular injection to be administered into the muscle in the buttock or thigh (see Baston et al 2009 for injection technique). However, Heelbeck (1999) reports a faster effect when the drug is given into the deltoid muscle of the arm (using a smaller needle), with therapeutic effect being achieved in 5 to 10 minutes rather than 20 minutes. Pethidine causes local irritation and repeated administration can lead to fibrosis of the muscle. The same site should not be used more than once during labour (Jordan 2002).

Effect on the woman

Heelbeck (1999) raises the issue that women who have been over-sedated in labour are unable to voice their wishes effectively. This can result in them agreeing to interventions or practices that they had previously felt quite strongly against. They may sleep for long periods and feel that they missed out on their labour experience. There is a fine balance between achieving analgesic effect and inducing drowsiness.

A lack of analgesic effect of both pethidine and other opioids administered to women in labour has been highlighted (Briker & Lavender 2002). Indeed, in one study (Olofsson et al 1996a) the authors concluded that it was unethical to meet women's requests for analgesia by sedating them. Another problem with pethidine use is the fact that professionals judge its effectiveness to be greater than the women who use it (Findley & Chamberlain 1999).

Although there are a range of hospital protocols for the administration of opioids during labour, in practice it often becomes common practice to use a standard dose, for example, 100 mg intramuscularly 3 to 4 hours apart. However, it may be more appropriate to use a smaller dose more frequently, depending on the needs of the individual woman. Larger doses of opioids are also associated with more nausea and vomiting (Maduska & Hajghassemali 1978). This can be prevented by administration of an anti-emetic, such as prochlorperazine (Stemetil) at the same time.

Respiratory depression is a side-effect of all opioids. Pethidine reduces the sensitivity of the respiratory centre to carbon dioxide. The rate and depth of breathing decreases and hypoxia may develop (Jordan 2002). It is essential to monitor a woman's respiratory rate closely following administration of pethidine, especially if she falls asleep.

The use of morphine in labour is less prevalent than the use of pethidine and is often restricted to women whose babies are known to have died in utero. It has a pronounced sedative effect but weak analgesic impact, although one study (Olofsson et al 1996b) did find a significant reduction in the experience of back pain with intravenous morphine.

Activity

Think about why opioids are not given orally during labour.

Find out the protocol for administration of pethidine to a labouring woman in the unit where you work.

Find out the usual dose for intramuscular prochlorperazine.

Revise the physiological control of respiration and the factors that impact on respiration rate.

Effect on the baby

Respiratory depression is also a problem for the neonate as pethidine passes across the placenta. The severity of respiratory depression varies depending on the dose to delivery interval as well as the total dose received. Elimination of pethidine is prolonged in the neonate as this process takes place in the liver, which is immature. The administration of opioids also leads to maternal bradycardia, which results in a drop in blood pressure. Placental perfusion may then be compromised, and a fetal bradycardia and loss of baseline variability of the fetal heart is often observed.

The opioid antagonist naloxone (Narcan neonatal) should always be nearby following administration of pethidine to a woman in labour. If the respiration rate of the neonate is depressed at birth, naloxone should be administered by the midwife immediately and further senior assistance called.

The neonate should be closely observed. S/he may require a repeat dose, as the half-life of naloxone is shorter than that of pethidine.

Activity

Find out the correct dose and route of administration of naloxone to a neonate with opioid-induced respiratory depression.

Identify which babies are particularly at risk of respiratory depression.

Find out about the policy where you work for caring for the neonate of a drug-dependent mother.

Breastfeeding

There is some evidence to suggest that administration of pethidine to a woman during labour is associated with an adverse effect on the future breastfeeding behaviour of the neonate (Rajan 1994, Nissen et al 1995, Ransjo-Arvidson et al 2001). In a study examining the effect of birth room practices on breastfeeding success (Righard & Alade 1990) it was reported that, of the neonates whose mothers had received pethidine during labour, 62% did not suck at all in the 2 hours following the birth.

Home birth

When a woman is anticipating a home birth she will discuss her analgesic requirements with the community midwife. In areas where the incidence of home birth is low, community midwives do not always carry a

supply of pethidine. If the woman requests pethidine, it can be supplied, via a prescription, from her general practitioner. As such, the pethidine is dispensed to the woman by a pharmacist and becomes her property.

Some GPs are reluctant to prescribe narcotics to pregnant women, being concerned that they will be responsible for its administration and effects. However, midwives can also obtain pethidine via a supply order from a supervisor of midwives (Department of Health 2007c) and dispensed by the hospital pharmacy. In the event that the pethidine is not used during the labour, the midwife must not destroy the drugs, as they remain the woman's property. She can advise the woman to destroy them in her presence or to return them to the pharmacist from which they were dispensed. The advice that is given and any subsequent action must be documented in the woman's records.

Epidural

An epidural in labour is a form of analgesia that involves the injection of a local anaesthetic into the epidural space. Larger doses can be given for instrumental or operative births. It involves the insertion of a small plastic catheter into the epidural space, through which drugs can be administered. In order to insert the plastic catheter, a Tuohy needle must first be carefully inserted through the skin and interspinous ligament by an anaesthetist (Fig. 6.1). The plastic catheter is then fed through the needle

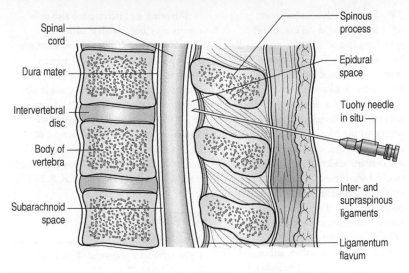

Spinal cord
Dura mater
Intervertebral disc
Body of vertebra
Subarachnoid space

Spinous process
Epidural space
Tuohy needle in situ
Inter- and supraspinous ligaments
Ligamentum flavum

Fig. 6.1 Sagittal section of the lumbar spine with Tuohy needle in the epidural space. (From Johnson & Taylor 2006, with permission.)

and the needle is then withdrawn, leaving the catheter in place. Once the epidural is in place, drugs can either be administered intermittently by a midwife, by continuous infusion or controlled by the woman (PCA). The provision of epidural services varies from unit to unit, and although many will provide a 24-hour service for labouring women, this is not a universal standard. In a large prospective study of women's expectations and experiences of childbirth (Green et al 2003) it was reported that women are increasingly wanting a pain-free labour: from 6% of primiparous women in 1987 to 21% in 2000. Women are also more likely to accept obstetric intervention generally (Green & Baston 2007).

Effect on the woman

Epidural analgesia is the most effective means of pain relief during labour and can bring welcome relief to women in labour. Unfortunately, this form of analgesia does not come without its disadvantages. The traditional high-dose epidural inhibits motor function and has been associated with increased operative delivery rates, longer labours and the need for labour to be augmented with oxytocin (Anim-Somuah 2005). However, one report suggests that low-dose epidurals and combined spinal epidurals (CSE) result in a higher spontaneous vaginal delivery rate (COMET 2001). This study reported a spontaneous vaginal delivery rate of

35% for the traditional epidural group, 43% for the low-dose, combined-spinal group and 43% for the low-dose infusion group. The CSE technique involves the use of a combination of low-dose opioid and local anaesthetic agents. The lower dose of local anaesthetic received reduces the impact on motor function associated with large doses via the traditional epidural route. A Cochrane review (Simmons et al 2007) of combined spinal-epidural versus traditional epidural analgesia in labour concluded that there was no difference between the two approaches for: mode of birth, maternal satisfaction, mobility or maternal hypotension, although CSE did provide faster onset of pain relief and less urinary retention.

In an attempt to reduce the risk of instrumental birth when epidural analgesia has been administered, some practitioners advocate discontinuing the epidural before the end of the first stage of labour. However a systematic review of the available research (Torvaldsen et al 2007) concluded that there was insufficient evidence to recommend this practice: no reduction in instrumental birth was demonstrated yet this practice was associated with an increase in inadequate pain relief during the second stage of labour.

Green et al (1998) found that satisfaction with the birth was related to how many drugs were used. They reported that the least satisfied women were those who used both pethidine and an epidural. The most satisfied women used nothing followed by those who used Entonox alone.

Shivering and itching are also side-effects associated with epidural use (Mayberry et al 2002). The woman may also need to have a urinary catheter inserted to empty her bladder as loss of sensation increases. Epidural use is also linked with maternal fever (Lieberman et al 1999) and associated infection screening postnatally (Lieberman & O'Donoghue 2002). Use of epidural analgesia during labour is not associated with long-term backache (NICE 2007).

Activity

Revise what a pudendal block is and when it is used.

Find out how a combined spinal epidural is administered.

Make sure you understand what is meant by the term 'intrathecal'.

Effect on the baby

Elevated maternal temperature leads to a rise in fetal temperature and hence an increased likelihood of being investigated and treated for potential infection. Epidurals have also been associated with hyperbilirubinaemia in neonates (Lieberman & O'Donoghue 2002); however, the cause of the association is unclear. Although epidural use is linked with increased instrumental delivery and oxytocin use (which are also associated with hyperbilirubinaemia), this does not explain the link found in all of the studies reported. CSE is reported to be associated with lower Apgar scores and the need for resuscitation, and this requires further exploration (COMET 2001).

Supporting the woman

For many women, the thought of having a needle inserted into her back is a daunting prospect. Having been informed of the potential risks and benefits of an epidural, the woman will also need information about what the procedure involves. The student midwife must learn how to provide this information in a way that is honest and clear, without causing unnecessary distress and fear. She must also include the birth partner and ensure that he or she is positioned to provide comfort to the woman, rather than witnessing the procedure.

Once the woman has made the decision and the midwife who is coordinating the delivery suite is aware of her request, the anaesthetist should be called without delay. As the procedure will take some time to perform and then further time for the drugs to work, the woman in established labour will continue to need support to cope with her labour pain. Entonox is particularly valuable at this time, combined with continuous support from the midwife.

Women receiving high-dose local anaesthetic drugs via an epidural catheter, such as bupivacaine, usually have an intravenous infusion started prior to its insertion. This is so that a bolus of fluids can be given to prevent maternal hypotension, which may lead to fetal heart rate anomalies. This has been shown to be beneficial when high-dose anaesthetic blocks are used but the evidence is unclear regarding the benefits in low-dose or combined spinal-epidural blocks (Hofmeyr et al 2004). In many maternity units, midwives have undertaken additional education and training to enable them to cannulate veins and provide continuity of carer.

Activity

Find out if midwives where you work undertake intravenous cannulation.

Research the evidence on prophylactic intravenous preloading for women who have low-dose local anaesthetics or opioid-only blocks via an epidural.

The woman will need to know that when the anaesthetist arrives s/he will ask her questions about her medical history and ask her to sign a consent form. She will be asked to curl herself around her baby, so that the spaces between her lumbar vertebrae increase to enable the needle to be positioned more easily. This is difficult for a pregnant woman to do and she will need help and encouragement. Some anaesthetists like the woman to be seated and to bend over, whereas others might ask her to curl up on her left side. The woman will need to bring her back to the edge of the bed and she will need reassurance that she is not going to fall off, but that this position helps the anaesthetist to obtain a clear view of her back. It is a sterile procedure so a pack of sterile equipment will be opened and the woman's back exposed and covered with a sterile cover with a hole through which the anaesthetist will work. Every effort must be made to maintain the woman's dignity.

As the anaesthetist will be working facing the woman's back, s/he may not be able to detect contractions. The student midwife can be the woman's advocate at this time, making it clear to the anaesthetist when a contraction is starting so that the procedure can stop for a short while and she can focus on supporting the woman through it. The fetal heart rate must be monitored throughout the procedure.

Activity

List the equipment required in the room when a woman has an epidural.

Consider what observations might lead you to suspect maternal hypotension. What emergency action would you take?

The woman will require advance warning that her back will be cleaned using a solution that feels cold. She will then feel some pressure as the anaesthetist uses his/her fingers to locate the correct position for insertion of the Tuohy needle. A local anaesthetic is then inserted into the skin of the back, typically described as a 'sharp scratch'. After this, the woman should not feel pain, but pressure and occasionally tingling as the needle and then the

catheter are put into position. Following this, the needle is removed and a filter is attached to the catheter, through which a test dose of the drug is administered. When the anaesthetist is confident that the catheter is in the correct place, the full dose is given and the sterile cover taken away so that the catheter can be taped to the woman's back.

It is then important that the woman is assisted to a comfortable position (never flat on her back). She will continue to feel her next couple of contractions, but they should gradually cease to be painful. The midwife will need to monitor the woman's blood pressure and pulse intensively following the procedure, in accordance with the anaesthetist's written instructions and/or local policy. The fetal heart rate and contractions must be recorded continuously following the insertion of a high-dose epidural block.

Midwives who have undertaken additional education and training and who have been assessed as competent are able to administer subsequent bolus or 'top-ups' to women, depending on local policy. Student midwives must not administer any drug via the epidural catheter.

A woman who has had a traditional epidural will become progressively more immobile with each subsequent bolus or top-up. She will not be able to change her own position and is dependent on her carers to ensure that her lower limbs do not fall off the bed as described by Thorpe et al (1990).

The loss of sensation of her lower limbs also means that the woman with an epidural in situ will not feel the discomfort normally experienced from being in the same position for too long. She becomes at high risk of developing pressure ulcers and will require regular position changes, immediate removal of soiled bedlinen and close observation of her skin for colour changes and abrasion.

 ## Reflection on trigger

Look back on the trigger scenario.

Siân is in active labour with her first baby. She has been using breathing and relaxation techniques but during her last contraction she asked for an epidural. Her partner looks shocked. Siân's birth plan states quite clearly that she does not plan to have one.

Now that you are familiar with pharmacological methods of pain relief you should have insight into how the scenario relates to the evidence about the issues. The jigsaw model will now be used to explore the trigger scenario in more depth.

Effective communication

It is clear from the scenario that Siân has previously communicated her intentions regarding the use of pain relief, both to her partner and to the midwife via her birth plan. It is useful if such communication happens before labour starts as it enables all involved to discuss the relative advantages and disadvantages of each method.

Questions that arise from the scenario might include: When did Siân decide that she would prefer not to have an epidural?

Did she discuss this with her midwife? Why is it important that Siân has discussed her hopes not to use an epidural with her partner? How can the partner reinforce Siân's hopes now? Should the midwife refer Siân to her birth plan at this stage or comply with her current request?

Woman-centred care

Where possible, care should be arranged to meet the requirements of the woman and reflect her aspirations for the birth. However, when a woman suddenly makes requests that are out of character with her previous intentions, every effort should be made to ensure that the midwife acts in her best interests. Questions that arise from the scenario might include: What strategies should the midwife employ in order to assess whether or not Siân would benefit from an epidural in the short and long term? What would you say to a woman who requests an epidural when she previously appeared to be coping well? Is it appropriate to involve the partner in the decision to have an epidural?

Using best evidence

Some women request an epidural towards the end of the first stage of labour because they are tired and cannot see an end to their pain. Women need feedback and information on which to base their decisions. If she had evidence that her cervix was almost fully dilated this may enable her to keep going without resorting to pharmacology. However, she may feel that she has had enough pain and look to the midwife to help resolve it. Questions that arise from the scenario might include: Why did Siân decide not to have an epidural? Does she know anyone who has used one? Does she know about the obstetric implications of having an epidural?

Professional and legal issues

The Code (NMC 2008:3) states that 'you must listen to the people in your care and respond to their concerns and preferences'. However, preferences can be difficult to judge when they change unexpectedly. Not to provide adequate analgesia to a woman who is requesting your support could be considered cruel and not acting in her best interests. Questions that arise from the scenario might include: Does the woman have capacity to consent to an epidural, when in the throes of advanced labour? Can the partner give consent on her behalf? How should this episode of care be documented?

Team working

During labour, the midwife, woman and her partner work together to achieve an optimum outcome. The midwife should work in partnership with them, involving them in decisions and providing information to help them choose options that best meet their individual needs. Questions that arise from the scenario might include: Who could the midwife consult for guidance regarding this issue? If the woman is adamant that an epidural is what she wants, which other members of the multi-professional team will be involved in her care? Can an epidural

service be provided 24 hours a day? In what circumstances would this not be possible?

Clinical dexterity

The midwife must respond to a woman's request for analgesia from a clinical as well as an empathetic perspective. She needs to take into account the whole clinical picture before she takes a particular course of action. She must use the clinical skills developed during her pre-registration programme but may also need to develop others that help enhance the care she can provide. Questions that arise from the scenario might include: If the woman requests an epidural, can the midwife cannulate a vein and commence an intravenous infusion? Has the midwife undertaken further training to enable her to administer further epidural top-up doses or manage a continuous infusion pump? Is she aware of the local guidelines for monitoring a woman with an epidural in situ?

Models of care

The scenario describes a woman in active labour. It does not state whether she is at home or in a hospital birthing room. The decisions she makes regarding pain relief in labour will influence the models of care she chooses. For example, epidural blocks are not available at home or in stand alone midwifery-led units; labour and birthing pools are not available in all consultant maternity units. Questions that arise from the scenario might include: Is Siân at home because she really did not want an epidural in labour?

Is Siân in hospital because she wanted to keep her options open about the type of pain relief she might use? How does the culture on the labour ward influence the way that midwives discuss options for pain relief with women?

Safe environment

The woman needs to feel safe and secure in the knowledge that the midwife will respond appropriately to her needs as they arise. She needs to know that the midwife is confident and competent to provide care in a safe and timely manner. Questions that arise from the scenario might include: How have the midwife's skills to care for a woman without the use of analgesia been assessed? Does the midwife feel confident to challenge the woman's request? Does she have the skills to help divert the woman from choosing an unecessary intervention? What additional observations would the midwife need to make if the woman had an epidural sited?

Promotes health

The midwife who cares for a woman in labour has the potential to influence the future health and wellbeing of the family unit. She can make a difference to how the woman looks back on her birth and contribute to this enduring memory. Questions that arise from the scenario might include: What are the potential health benefits of having an epidural in labour? How might having an epidural impact on Siân's future physical and mental health? If Siân has

an epidural, how will this impact on the baby? How would an epidural influence her postnatal recovery?

Further scenarios

The following scenarios enable you to consider how specific situations influence the care the midwife provides. Use the jigsaw model to explore the issues raised in the scenario.

Scenario 1

Reesha has had pethidine to help her relax during her labour. She is now sleeping and does not seem to be aware of her surroundings. She suddenly opens her eyes and says, 'I think I'm going to be sick.'

Practice point

Not all women respond to pethidine in the same way: some become very sleepy and others do not feel that it has much effect. It is difficult to predict the response unless they have had the drug before. One of the common side-effects of all narcotics is nausea and vomiting.

Further questions specific to Scenario 1 include:

1. Did Reesha know about the side-effects of pethidine before she asked for or consented to its administration?

2. How could the side-effects of nausea and vomiting be minimized?

3. Does pethidine have other unwanted side-effects?

4. Could Reesha enter the pool for birth having had pethidine?

5. What clinical observations should the midwife make following administration of pethidine?

6. What adptations to the physical environments should be made when a woman is very drowsy following the use of pethidine?

Scenario 2

Liz is at home in active labour. At the last vaginal assessment, her cervix was approximately 8 cm dilated. She is finding each contraction more difficult to cope with and is finding it hard to focus on her breathing, despite the attentions of her partner. The midwife says, 'Have you thought about trying some Entonox?'

Practice point

Entonox is a useful substance for helping women relax and reduce the feelings of panic when contractions become difficult to bear. Of particular value is its means of administration: having to breathe deeply to activate the release of the nitrous oxide and oxygen mixture helps some women to re-focus and regain control. However, it does not have the same impact on all women and some find it has the opposite effect, leading them to feel light-headed and not engaged with the situation.

Resources

Association of Radical Midwives: Analgesia: meptid versus pethidine. http://www.radmid.demon.co.uk/meptid.htm.

Further questions specific to Scenario 2 include:

1. What pain relief had Liz considered for use at home?

2. Should the midwife make suggestions about alternative analgesia or wait until the woman asks?

3. Do all community midwives carry Entonox?

4. How long does a cylinder last?

5. How can it be replenished if it runs out?

6. Does the use of Entonox in the home pose any risks for the midwives present at the birth?

7. What precautions should the midwife take when transporting Entonox in her car?

Conclusion

The search for the ideal method of analgesia in labour has a long way to go. Each method has advantages and disadvantages that need exploring and considering antenatally, before analgesia is required. The midwife has a sensitive role to play in presenting the facts to women in a way that is truthful but not alarmist. Women need to be aware of all methods as their circumstances and requirements may change.

Breastfeeding Mums: Pain relief in labour: gas and air. http://www.breastfeedingmums.com/Pain-Relief-During-Childbirth-Gas-and-Air.htm.

NHS Direct: What are my pain relief options during labour?. http://www.nhsdirect.nhs.uk/articles/article.aspx?articleId=914.

NHS Direct: Will an epidural help during labour?. http://www.nhsdirect.nhs.uk/articles/article.aspx?articleid=915.

References

Anim-Somuah M, Smyth R, Howell C: Epidural versus non-epidural or no analgesia in labour DOI: 10.1002/14651858.CD000331.pub2, *Cochrane Database of Systematic Reviews* 3(CD000331), 2005.

Arfeen Z, Armstrong P, Whitfield A: The effects of Entonox and epidural analgesia on arterial oxygen saturation of women in labour, *Anaesthesia* 49(1):32–34, 1994.

Baston H, Hall J, Henley-Einion: *Midwifery essentials: basics*, Edinburgh, 2009, Elsevier.

BOC: Gases data sheet (Nitrous oxide). Last revised. January 12, 1999. Online. Available http://www1.boc.com/uk/sds/. December 10, 2008.

Briker L, Lavender T: Parenteral opioids for labor pain relief: a systematic review, *American Journal of Obstetrics and Gynecology* 186(5):S94–S109, 2002.

COMET: Effect of low-dose mobile versus traditional epidural techniques on mode of delivery: a randomised controlled trial. Comparative Obstetric Mobile Epidural Trial (COMET) Study Group UK, *Lancet* 358(9275):19–23, 2001.

Department of Health: *Making it better: for mother and baby*, Clinical case for change (Shribman). London, 2007a, Department of Health.

Department of Health: *Maternity matters: choice, access and continuity of care in a safe service*, London, 2007b, Department of Health.

Department of Health: *Safer management of controlled drugs. A guide to good practice in secondary care (England)*, London, 2007c, Department of Health.

Findley I, Chamberlain G: ABC of labour care. Relief of pain, *British Medical Journal* 318:927–930, 1999.

Green J, Coupland V, Kitzinger J: *Great expectations. A prospective study of women's expectations and experiences of childbirth*, Hale, 1998, Books for Midwives.

Green J, Baston H, Easton S, et al: *Greater expectations? Inter-relationships between expectations and experiences of decision making, continuity, choice and control in labour, and psychological outcomes*, Leeds, 2003, University of Leeds, Mother & Infant Research Unit.

Green JM, Baston HA: Have women become more willing to accept obstetric interventions and does this relate to mode of birth? Data from a prospective study, *Birth* 34(1):6–13, 2007.

Heelbeck L: Administration of pethidine in labour, *British Journal of Midwifery* 7(6):372–377, 1999.

Hofmeyr GJ, Cyna AM, Middleton P: Prophylactic intravenous preloading for regional analgesia in labour DOI: 10.1002/14651858.CD000175.pub2, *Cochrane Database of Systematic Reviews* 2(CD000175), 2004.

Johnson R, Taylor W: *Skills for midwifery practice*, ed 2, Edinburgh, 2006, Elsevier.

Jordan S: *Pharmacology for midwives – the evidence base for safe practice*, Basingstoke, 2002, Palgrave.

Lieberman E, Cohen A, Lang C, et al: Maternal intrapartum temperature elevation as a risk factor for cesarean delivery and assisted vaginal delivery, *American Journal of Public Health* 89:506–510, 1999.

Lieberman E, O'Donoghue C: Unintended effects of epidural analgesia during labour: a systematic review, *American Journal of Obstetrics and Gynecology* 186(5):S31–S68, 2002.

Maduska A, Hajghassemali A: A double-blind comparison of butophanol and meperidine in labour: maternal pain relief and effect on the newborn, *Canadian Anaesthetist's Society Journal* 25(5):398–404, 1978.

Maternity Care Working Party: *Making normal birth a reality. Consensus statement from the Maternity Care Working Party (MCWP)*, London, 2007, MCWP.

Mayberry L, Clemmens D, De A: Epidural analgesia side effects, co-interventions, and care of women during childbirth: a systematic review, *American Journal of Obstetrics and Gynecology* 186(5):S81–S93, 2002.

Misuse of Drugs Regulations, 2001. http://www.opsi.gov.uk/si/si2001/20013998.htm.

National Institute for Health and Clinical Excellence (NICE): *Intrapartum care. Care of healthy women and their babies during childbirth. NICE clinical guideline 55*, London, 2007, NICE.

Nissen E, Lilja G, Matthiesen A, et al: Effects of maternal pethidine on infants' developing breastfeeding behaviour, *Acta Paediatrica* 84(2):140–145, 1995.

Nursing and Midwifery Council (NMC): *Standards for medicines management*, London, 2007, NMC.

Nursing and Midwifery Council (NMC): *The Code. Standards of conduct, performance and ethics for nurse and midwives*, London, 2008, NMC.

Olofsson C, Ekblom A, Ekman-Ordeberg G, et al: Lack of analgesic effect of systemically administered morphine or pethidine on labour pain, *British Journal of Obsterics and Gynaecology* 103(10):968–972, 1996a.

Olofsson C, Ekblom A, Ekman-Ordeberg G, et al: Analgesic efficacy of intravenous morphine on labour pain: a reappraisal, *International Journal of Obstetric Anesthesia* 5(3):176–180, 1996b.

Rajan L: The impact of obstetric procedures and analgesia/anaesthesia during labour and delivery on breastfeeding, *Midwifery* 10(2): 87–103, 1994.

Ransjo-Arvidson A, Mathieson A, Lilja G, et al: Maternal analgesia during labor disturbs newborn behavior: effects on breastfeeding, temperature and crying, *Birth* 28(1):5–12, 2001.

Righard L, Alade M: Effect of delivery room routines on success of first breastfeed, *Lancet* 336(8723): 1105–1107, 1990.

Simmons SW, Cyna AM, Dennis AT, et al: Combined spinal-epidural versus epidural analgesia in labour DOI: 10.1002/14651858.CD003401.pub2, *Cochrane Database of Systematic Reviews* 2(CD003401), 2007.

The Health Act, 2006. Online. Available http://www.opsi.gov.uk/acts/acts2006/pdf/ukpga_20060028_en.pdf.

Thorpe J, McNitt J, Leppert P: Effects of epidural analgesia: some questions and answers, *Birth* 17(3):157–162, 1990.

Torvaldsen S, Roberts CL, Bell JC, et al: Discontinuation of epidural analgesia late in labour for reducing the adverse delivery outcomes associated with epidural analgesia DOI: 10.1002/14651858.CD004457.pub2, *Cochrane Database of Systematic Reviews* 4(CD004457), 2007.

Chapter 7

Induced or accelerated labour

Trigger scenario

It is 9.30 p.m. and Isobel is alone. She has had some prostaglandin gel more than 1 hour ago as she is now 2 weeks overdue. Her partner was asked to leave the ward at 9 p.m. and the monitor was disconnected shortly after that. But the midwife was called away by a distant buzzer, and now Isobel doesn't know what to do. Can she get up? Should she ring her buzzer? They all seem so busy.

Introduction

A large proportion of women experience induction of labour. More than 20% of women in England underwent this procedure during 2005–6 (The Information Centre 2007). Usually invasive, and often resulting in additional discomfort, this intervention must be managed with care and sensitivity. Student midwives need to develop an understanding of the indications for induction and acceleration of labour, the underlying principles and potential consequences. This chapter aims to address some of the most salient issues, with particular emphasis on providing woman-focused care.

Induction of labour

The National Institute for Health and Clinical Excellence (NICE), in its clinical guideline (NICE 2008:xii), defined induction of labour as 'the artificial initiation of labour'. The rates of induction and augmentation of labour have significant geographical variation (Williams et al 1998). Also, despite the publication of NICE guidance (NICE 2001, 2008) with the aim of supporting evidence-based care, a wide variation in current practice continues.

Investigation in this area of obstetric practice is complex because of the many variables that can potentially combine. Not only are there many ways in which induction of labour can be attempted – for example, with prostaglandin preparations – but there is also a range of doses and routes of administration. The rationale for induction of labour, gestation of the pregnancy and favourability of the cervix are additional considerations that need to be taken into account when examining the literature.

Reasons for inducing labour

Post-maturity

The risk of stillbirth and neonatal mortality increases with post-maturity. In a large retrospective analysis of birth outcomes and subsequent survival to 1 year (Hilder et al 1998), it was found that the risk of stillbirth increases six times from 0.35 per 1000 total births at 37 weeks' gestation to 2.12 per 1000 at 43 weeks' gestation. Following a systematic review of the evidence (Gülmezoglu et al 2006) it was concluded that routine induction of labour after 41 weeks' gestation improves perinatal mortality compared to waiting for spontaneous labour. Induction of labour is therefore recommended between 41 and 42 weeks' gestation (NICE 2008).

Not all women wish to accept intervention, and would rather wait and see what happens. Heimstad et al (2007) conducted a randomized controlled trial to determine the outcome of expectant management with serial fetal surveillance (every third day) versus induction of labour at 41 weeks' gestation. There were no significant differences between the two groups with

regard to mode of birth or neonatal morbidity. Women in the induction group were more likely to have a precipitate birth and a shorter second stage of labour.

However, a study designed to determine the cost-effectiveness of induction of labour versus serial monitoring while awaiting spontaneous labour reported an increase in caesarean section in the expectant group (Goeree et al 1995). There were no differences in perinatal mortality, but the cost of expectant management was greater because of the increased rate of caesarean. NICE guidance (2008) recommends that serial monitoring should be initiated at 42 weeks, for women who decline induction of labour, and should include twice-weekly cardiotocography and ultrasound estimation of the single deepest pool of liquor.

Pathology

The benefits of induction of labour must be carefully weighed against the potential hazards. Where maternal or fetal pathology exists or is suspected, the outcome may benefit if the pregnancy were brought to a swift conclusion.

Activity

List three maternal and three fetal indications for induction of labour.

Ruptured membranes

NICE guidance (2007) recommends that woman who have pre-labour ruptured membranes should be offered induction of labour approximately 24 hours after the membranes had ruptured. The guidelines go on to state that if a woman chooses to await events for more than 24 hours she should record her temperature every 4 hours whilst awake and report any change in the colour of her vaginal loss. In a rare survey of women's views about induction, Hodnett et al (1997) compared women's preferences for induction of labour or expectant management in women with pre-labour rupture of membranes at term. Women in the induction group were less likely to report additional worry, or that there was nothing they liked about the treatment, than women in the expectant group.

Mental health

In rare circumstances, a woman may be so fearful about going into labour that induction provides a welcome alternative to escalating anxiety and distress. Such intervention enables the labour to progress in a more controlled pattern, and care to be provided by a known midwife. The woman's care should also be planned in liaison with the mental health team so that a psychiatric assessment can be undertaken. Women who are anxious antenatally require careful monitoring and support in the postnatal period as they are more likely to go on to suffer from postnatal depression (Areskog et al 1984).

Social

Occasionally, it becomes necessary to expedite birth due to extenuating social circumstances. Examples of such situations include: partners of servicemen who are only allowed fixed leave from duty; single women who have limited support from family or friends and for whom the birth can be arranged to fit in with special arrangements; and the terminal illness of a close friend or relative. Each case must be judged on its own merits, and the woman must be carefully informed about the associated risks. NICE (2008) recommend that induction for maternal request is audited.

Contraindications to induction of labour

Induction of labour should not be attempted where there is placenta praevia, transverse or oblique lie and/or suspected cephalopelvic disproportion. Induction should not be considered if there is evidence of severe fetal growth restriction with confirmed fetal compromise (NICE 2008).

A woman who has had a previous caesarean section has a scar on her uterus; extreme caution is therefore essential when induction of labour is being considered. An American study (Sims et al 2001) was conducted to determine the safety and success of trial of labour in women who were induced compared with those who had a spontaneous labour. It found that women whose labour was induced were less likely to achieve a vaginal delivery (58% compared with 77% in the spontaneous labour group), and that 7% had separation of the uterine scar. They concluded that induction of labour in women aiming for vaginal birth after caesarean section is associated with a significant risk of serious maternal morbidity.

Impact of induction of labour

Induction of labour has been shown to impact on the subsequent mode of birth. In a retrospective cohort study of 14 409 women, induction of labour increased the risk of caesarean section for both primiparous and multiparous women, independent of other risk factors such as maternal and gestational age (Heffner et al 2003). Having made the decision that delivery is the best course of action, failing to induce labour may also result in emergency caesarean section.

With this adverse consequence in mind, it is important that the most effective means of inducing labour are employed. Current practice involves activities to prime or ripen the cervix prior to instigating further interventions. The use of some of the methods and preparations available will now be described.

Methods of induction

Cervical priming

In the last weeks of pregnancy the cervix begins to soften and efface (ripen). This process is enhanced if the presenting part of the fetus and forewaters are well applied to the cervix as this pressure will increase the release of local prostaglandins. Cervical priming is an intervention with the aim of stimulating uterine activity and speeding up the ripening process.

The ripeness of the cervix is assessed during vaginal examination. One way of describing the consistency of the cervix that is sometimes used to help students is to compare the consistency of your nose (firm) with that of your lips (soft). Bishop (1964) developed a score to make this assessment more objective, a summary of which is given in Table 7.1. Each aspect of the assessment is given a score, and the total of all five aspects is the 'Bishop's score'. An unfavourable cervix (for induction of labour) has a Bishop's score of four or less, whereas women whose cervices have a score of eight or more have the same chance of vaginal delivery as someone who went into spontaneous labour (Chamberlain & Zander 1999).

Interventions for cervical priming and induction of labour

Membrane sweep

This technique is employed with the intention of hastening the onset of regular uterine contractions. It is performed during vaginal examination and involves insertion of a finger through the cervical os and, in a circular movement, separating the amnion from the lower uterine segment. This procedure is sometimes accompanied by an additional stretching of the uterine os by the examiner's fingers and is then termed 'stretch and sweep' (Fig. 7.1).

Table 7.1 Summary of Bishop's score assessment

	0	1	2	3
Position of cervix	Posterior	mid-position	anterior	–
Consistency of cervix	Firm	Medium	Soft	–
Cervical length or effacement	3 cm not effaced	2 cm partially effaced	1 cm almost effaced	0 cm fully effaced
Station of presenting part (cm above ischial spines)	3 cm above	2 cm above	0–1 cm above	Below ischial spines
Dilation of the cervix	0 cm	1–2 cm	3–4 cm	5–6 cm

Implementation of this procedure has been somewhat ad hoc, with some practitioners offering it to all women who return to the antenatal clinic after their expected date of birth. Others have taken the view that it is an uncomfortable procedure that may lead to bleeding, pre-labour rupture of membranes and irregular contractions. A systematic review of membrane sweeping for induction of labour concluded that, although the procedure did reduce the need for induction of labour by drugs, this advantage should be carefully weighed against potential for discomfort and unpleasant side-effects (Boulvain et al 2004). However, the NICE (2008) guidance advocates that this procedure should be offered to nulliparous women when reviewed after 40 weeks' gestation and all women at 41 weeks' gestation. It is therefore essential that women are informed of the potential side-effects as well as the advantages to enable them to make a decision that is right for them.

Mechanical methods

The first methods for inducing labour were mechanical and although not currently in widespread use their effectiveness has been explored in a systematic review (Boulvain et al 2001). The methods reviewed included catheters inflated in the cervical canal and laminaria tents. The review concluded that there is insufficient evidence to recommend their use although compared with the use of oxytocin in women whose cervix was

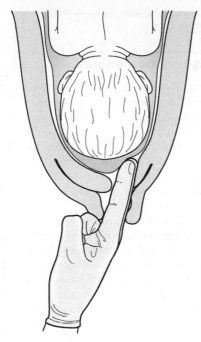

Fig. 7.1 Sweeping the membranes. (From Johnson & Taylor 2006, with permission.)

not favourable, mechanical methods were associated with a lower casearean section rate.

Prostaglandin E2 (PGE2)

PGE2 is an effective agent for ripening the cervix (D'Aniello et al 2003). It is available in either tablet, gel or pessary form, all of which, according to a systematic review (Kelly et al 2003), appear to be as efficacious as each other. The authors also concluded that lower dose regimens (total dose of less than

or equal to 3 mg) appear as efficacious as higher dose regimens (total dose of more than 3 mg).

NICE guidance (2008) recommends that either PGE2 vaginal tablets, gel or slow release pessary should be used as the method of preference. Doses of PGE2 tablets or gel can be repeated every 6 hours (maximum two doses) whereas only one dose of slow release PGE2 should be given in 24 hours. Intravenous, extra-amniotic, intracervical or oral PGE2 is not recommended for induction of labour (NICE 2008).

Activity

Find out about the following non-pharmacological methods described to induce labour: acupuncture, nipple stimulation, enema, foley catheter.
Find out if your mentor has cared for women using alternative methods of induction of labour and, if so, whether they were successful.

Care: First impressions

Historically, women have sometimes been admitted to an antenatal/postnatal ward in the evening for vaginal PGE2 with the aim of having artificial rupture of membranes and successful induction of labour the following day. However, NICE guidelines recommend that induction should commence in the morning as this is associated with enhanced client satisfaction (NICE 2008). When a woman is admitted to the maternity unit for induction of labour, it is particularly important that she feels treated as an individual. To be greeted in a way that acknowledges that her arrival was expected is an important first step. Showing her to her bed bay with her name already displayed can help convey this. Her hospital notes should already be on the ward. Some women will go into spontaneous labour before they reach the antenatal ward; for this reason, some units do not make preparations for their arrival so as not to 'waste time'. However, to be expected and to have this demonstrated in whatever small level of preparedness can build the woman's confidence in the system.

Some maternity units have a specially allocated induction suite. This can help women to be cared for in an environment where care is focused on particular needs rather than shared between women who are ill or who have already had their babies.

One issue that is often difficult to manage is if the woman's partner has to leave shortly after the prostaglandin has been administered. This is a time when the woman may feel vulnerable and alone, not sure when to ask for attention or what the long night might hold. Some induction facilities enable partners to stay overnight using a put-up bed, thus providing a family-focused approach to care.

If your unit has a policy that enables women to return home after administration of PGE2 she should be asked to contact the midwife if she does not have any contractions after 6 hours

or when contractions begin (NICE 2008).

Admission procedure

The documentary side of this process will have common elements to any admission to the ward. However, the woman need not be aware that you have undertaken the same process three times already that day. She needs to feel that you are focused on her and that you are making efforts to get to know her and her unique circumstances.

The student can make a huge difference to the woman's experience. You will need to identify what she likes to be called, and then tell her your name and how long you will be caring for her. If you are working an evening shift, she might be disappointed that you will soon be going off-duty, but reassured to hear that you will be back the following morning and anticipate continuing to care for her then. Many maternity units encourage students to follow women through the process of induction as part of the learning process. If you have been caring for someone undergoing induction, it is worth asking the midwife in charge if you can go with the woman to the labour ward – even if you are unable to stay all shift. This will help the woman acclimatize to her new environment and carers with someone she trusts at her side. Such continuity may not always be possible, either due to staff shortages or organizational problems. The student should not make any promises that she may not be able to keep as this could lead to disappointment and a breakdown in trust. If you say to her that you will come and visit her on the postnatal ward when she has had the baby, she will be hoping that you do.

Monitoring the fetal heart rate

Prior to administration of vaginal PGE2 a normal fetal heart rate pattern should be confirmed using electronic fetal monitoring (NICE 2008). Subsequent to administration of PGE2 the fetal heart shold be monitored electronically, when contractions begin. If a normal pattern is observed, intermittent auscultation can be the method of choice.

Administration of PGE2

This should only be undertaken by a midwife following the provision of a dated, timed and signed prescription and under the written instruction and (indirect) supervision of a doctor. Local policy should provide clear guidance for the midwife who performs this role, giving clear parameters within which she can practise and when she should seek medical advice. Two qualified midwives should check the drugs and identity of the woman. The woman should be reminded of the procedure and be able to give consent. Privacy and dignity must be maintained, and an abdominal palpation and CTG undertaken immediately prior to its administration. The procedure involves that followed during normal vaginal examination (Chapter 3), with insertion of the prostaglandin into the posterior fornix of the vagina.

If cervical priming is successful, artificial rupture of the membranes (ARM) will become possible, as the cervix becomes sufficiently central and dilated.

It is not part of the midwife's role to perform ARM on a woman who is not in active labour. This is the doctor's role. However, if the woman starts having regular, painful uterine contractions, and her cervix effaces and dilates, then ARM can be undertaken by the midwife with the woman's consent. Amniotomy alone (without cervical ripening or in the absence of uterine contractions) is not advocated as a means of inducing labour (Bricker & Lukas 2000).

Oxytocin

Oxytocin, a hormone secreted from the posterior pituitary gland, causes contraction of smooth muscle. The uterine muscle (myometrium) has oxytocin receptors which increase in number towards the end of pregnancy. Following cervical ripening and ARM the uterus may still be reluctant to contract regularly and effectively. Synthetic oxytocin can be administered to work in addition to the woman's own endogenous production to increase the contractility of the uterus.

When the membranes are ruptured, either artificially or spontaneously, oxytocin can be administered via an intravenous infusion, following written instruction from a doctor. However, oxytocin should not be commenced within 6 hours of administration of

PGE2. An intravenous infusion will need to be sited, and all fluids and additives carefully checked and labelled, by a qualified midwife. During its administration, uterine activity and the fetal heart rate must be continuously monitored. Oxytocin must be given via an infusion pump so that it can be carefully titrated against uterine activity. The aim with an oxytocin infusion is to achieve three to four contractions in 10 minutes, and this may be achieved before the maximum dose is reached.

The treatment regime is written in milliunits per minute (mU/min) and is increased every 30 minutes, from 1 mU/min up to a maximum licensed dose of 20 mU/min, over 3 hours (NICE 2001). Meticulous documentation of uterine activity and dosage of oxytocin administered must be maintained. Oxytocin should not be used either alone or with amniotomy (Howarth & Botha 2001) as the primary means of inducing labour unless there is a contraindication to the use of PGE2 (NICE 2008).

Activity

List the side-effects of intravenous oxytocin.

Revise how you would recognize fetal compromise, and what would be your first three actions.

Misoprostol and induction of labour

Misoprotol is a prostaglandin used to ripen the cervix prior to medical and surgical termination of pregnancy. It is currently unlicensed for use for induction of labour. However, there is much debate in the professional press regarding its use for this purpose.

Vaginal misoprostol has been associated with hyperstimulation of the uterus (Fisher et al 2001). However, Goldberg & Wing (2003) recommend its use in low doses (vaginally) in situations where the woman can be carefully monitored. A systematic review of the use of vaginal misoprostol for cervical ripening and induction of labour (Hofmeyr & Gülmezoglu 2003) concluded that the studies available for review were not large enough to exclude serious adverse events, such as uterine rupture.

The MisoPROM study (Mozurkewich et al 2003) compared women who had labour induced with oral misoprostol with those who had intravenous oxytocin, focusing primarily on caesarean section rates. They found no difference between the two groups for caesarean section rates or length of time to vaginal delivery, although those receiving misoprostol had fewer postpartum haemorrhages.

However, Beigi et al (2003) found that, when used for cervical ripening in women with a Bishop's score of five or less, a single dose of oral misoprostol significantly reduced the rate of caesarean section compared with a placebo. Interventions that have the potential to reduce the rising casearean rate are likely to be explored further.

Another drug, mifepristone, has also been considered for induction of labour. A systematic review (Neilson 2000) concluded that there is insufficient evidence to recommend its use although there was an apparent reduction in caesarean births when used for induction which would warrant its consideration in future research trials. NICE guidelines (2008) do not recommend the use of either misoprostol or mifepristone to women with a live fetus.

Activity

Find out how much each of these methods of induction costs.

Find out what is meant by the terms 'uterine tachysystole' and 'uterine hypersystole'.

Pain relief

Induction of labour can be difficult to cope with, and many factors need to be considered before choices are made. Hopefully, the woman will have had information at her local maternity unit about the options available to her before she is distracted by painful contractions. If she has made a decision this may need to be reviewed in the light of impending induction of labour. NICE recommends that the woman is informed that her labour may be more painful than spontaneous labour (NICE 2008). It is difficult to say how long it will take to induce labour, and this delay may be a contributory factor in how able the woman is to cope with contractions. She may have been unable to sleep or rest due to her strange environment and separation from family. Irregular contractions and the excitement that they might soon progress into the real thing may also have disturbed her. Although an epidural might bring welcome rest, it has to be considered in the light of increased risk of instrumental delivery (Lieberman & O'Donoghue 2002).

If the woman wishes to avoid pharmacological methods of analgesia, she will need a lot of support. The midwife can also act as her advocate, by suggesting to the doctor who wants to perform ARM and start Syntocinon at the same time, that perhaps the latter could be delayed while the woman becomes acclimatized to a sudden burst of uterine activity.

The use of water in labour is not contraindicated and is recommended by the NICE Guidelines (2008:13).

Acceleration of labour

Sometimes labour starts spontaneously but then slows down or stops. Alternatively, contractions may remain frequent but are short in duration or weak in strength. If the woman is able to be mobile in labour, such a slowdown can sometimes be reversed by becoming more upright and active. The presenting part becomes more applied to the cervix, and contractions are stimulated again. If the woman has intact membranes, she may request to have them ruptured with the aim of stimulating further contractions. A stretch and sweep might be suggested. In the absence of fetal compromise, she may prefer to await events and be glad of the rest. Delay in the first stage of labour is diagnosed if cervical dilatation is less than 2 cm in 4 hours (NICE 2007).

Activity

Consider the national maternity record. This document includes sections that prompt the woman to ask questions about how her care may be managed. For example, the section 'slow progress in labour' includes questions such as: 'Why might labour be slow?', 'Why might a Syntocinon drip be suggested?'. Think about how you would answer such enquiries.

Occasionally, a woman makes excellent progress throughout labour but a rim or lip of cervix remains – preventing her from progressing to the second stage of labour. She may require an oxytocin infusion and epidural to help conclude dilatation and prevent her from pushing against the cervix during transition. This can be a huge disappointment for her, and she will need lots of encouragement and praise for her efforts.

Another scenario could be that regular painful contractions continue but the cervix is slow to dilate. The senior midwife should be informed of 'failure to progress' during the active phase of labour. The doctor will be asked to review the situation and will seek your description of current progress prior to making his/her assessment. This will involve performing a vaginal examination to confirm the dilatation

of the cervix and identification of the position of the presenting part.

Malposition can lead to incoordinate uterine action, and may be corrected with an oxytocin infusion. The woman should continue to be involved in all decisions about her care, and be able to make judgments based on the information she receives.

Activity

What might lead you to suspect that the fetus was in the occipito-posterior position? Consider what additional support the woman might require from you.

A woman requiring augmentation for a prolonged labour will probably value an epidural for pain relief. She will be tired, and an epidural may allow her to get some rest so that she can enjoy the arrival of her new baby.

Reflection on trigger

Look back on the trigger scenario.

It is 9.30 p.m. and Isobel is alone. She has had some prostaglandin gel more than 1 hour ago as she is now 2 weeks overdue. Her partner was asked to leave the ward at 9 p.m. and the monitor was disconnected shortly after that. But the midwife was called away by a distant buzzer, and now Isobel does not know what to do. Can she get up? Should she ring her buzzer? They all seem so busy.

Now that you are familiar with the principles of induction of labour you should have insight into how the scenario relates to the issues involved. The jigsaw model will now be used to explore the trigger scenario in more depth.

Effective communication

It is clear from the scenario that there has been a failure of communication. Midwives are often so familiar with the practices of the maternity unit that they fail to communicate what the woman can expect to happen to her over the course of her care. When women are left alone, particularly after visiting hours, they can feel very vulnerable and isolated. Questions that arise from the scenario might include: Did Isobel receive any written information prior to admission for induction of her labour? Has there been a handover of shift that has left Isobel in the gap between what one midwife thinks the other will do and what the other midwife thinks has already been done? How can communication between women and their carers be enhanced during this very common procedure?

Woman-centred care

Women who are admitted to hospital for induction of labour should feel that they are the focus of attention, that they were expected and that the arrival of their new baby is the central concern of all involved. Even though the woman requires this intervention in order to get labour started, this does not mean that she must relinquish all her hopes and plans for labour. Questions that arise from the scenario might include: What can the midwives do to ensure that the process of labour and birth still remains one in which Isobel makes decisions and feels involved in her care? How can the experience be personalized for Isobel? Does she have a named midwife responsible for her particular needs?

Using best evidence

When an intervention as purposeful as induction of labour is recommended, women need to know that it is the most appropriate course of action in her individual circumstances. Questions that arise from the scenario might include: Is prostaglandin gel the most effective method of inducing labour for post-maturity? What evidence is there to support admitting someone to hospital and then administering prostaglandin at night rather than during the day? Has Isobel had a membrane sweep by the community midwife? Are there any other equally effective methods of inducing labour? Are there clear local guidelines that support midwifery practice in relation to induction of labour? If so, do they reflect national guidelines?

Professional and legal issues

Although it may not be a requirement that women give written consent for induction of labour, they need to understand the risks and benefits in order to give informed consent. Midwives must only provide care that they have been trained in and need to acknowledge the limits of their professional role. Questions that arise from the scenario might include: Does the midwife understand the process by which prostaglandins work and their potential side-effects? How is the prostaglandin prescribed? Where is its administration documented? Which professional is responsible for gaining consent from the woman to induce her labour? What would the midwife do if the woman had declined induction of labour?

Team working

The midwife's role and sphere of practice is normal childbirth. She continues to care for women who require intervention, in cooperation with other members of the maternity care team. The midwife must take account of the whole picture when initiating a process that, once started, must be followed through. Questions that arise from the scenario might include: What is the activity on the rest of the maternity unit? Can this woman be closely observed and cared for within the current workload? Whom should the midwife liaise with before induction of labour is commenced? Who has overall responsibility for Isobel's care?

Clinical dexterity

Being able to initiate induction of labour requires the midwife to be able to undertake abdominal palpation, vaginal examination and commence continuous electronic fetal monitoring. She needs to perform these skills with confidence and have the knowledge and understanding

to interpret what she finds. Questions that arise from the scenario might include: How did the midwife learn to administer prostaglandin gel? Who supervised her? How does the midwife maintain her skills? How often does she care for women during the antenatal and intrapartum period? What opportunities does she have to learn from and share her own skills and knowledge with others?

Models of care

Induction of labour is only practised in a hospital environment in this country. Thus if a woman had previously wanted a home birth and then does not go into labour within 42 weeks' gestation, she is likely to be encouraged to come into hospital. Similarly, if a woman had hoped to give birth in a midwifery-led unit, she is likely to fall outside their admission criteria if she needs induction of labour. Questions that arise from the scenario might include: Is hospital the most appropriate place for induction of labour? What are the advantages and disadvantages of being in hospital from early labour until the birth?

Safe environment

With relation to all aspects of healthcare, patient safety is high on the government's agenda (Department of Health 2006). Healthcare workers are encouraged to report risks and take actions that enable them to learn from mistakes. Questions that arise from the scenario might include: What midwifery care will Isobel need during the night? Could induction of labour be safely carried out in the home environment? What are the potential risks and benefits of undertaking this procedure at home? Is it safe for Isobel to walk around following insertion of prostoglandin gel? What action would be taken if the midwife had used the wrong dose of prostaglandin?

Promotes health

It can take hours for induction of labour to be successful and regular uterine contractions to become established. During this waiting time the midwife can encourage the woman to use distraction techniques, to remain active when awake yet to maximize opportunities to get plenty of rest. Questions that arise from the scenario might include: How can the midwife help Isobel maintain a positive attitude and faith in her body to birth her baby? What are the risks associated with bed rest and how can women take active steps to reduce those risks?

Further scenarios

The following scenarios enable you to consider how specific situations influence the care the midwife provides. Use the jigsaw model to explore the issues raised in each scenario.

Scenario 1

Caroline has been in labour with her first baby for 12 hours. Her cervix has been 6 cm dilated for the last 2 hours and her contractions have become less frequent. The midwife suggests that she might need 'a little help' and asks the registrar if she can commence a Syntocinon infusion.

Practice point

There are many reasons that might account for Caroline's apparent 'delay in first stage'. Syntocinon via intravenous infusion is one method of accelerating a slow labour, but there are other alternatives that the midwife could try, including encouraging her to change position, ensuring that her bladder is not full and taking her for a walk.

Further questions specific to Scenario 1 include:

1. Has the midwife tried any alternative approaches to labour acceleration before considering Syntocinon?
2. What do the local guidelines say about delay in the first stage of labour?
3. If the fetal heart rate is satisfactory and the woman is content, why does labour require 'a little help'?
4. Who can commence Syntocinon infusions?
5. Has the midwife explained the risks and benefits to Caroline?
6. What observations should the midwife undertake on Caroline if she agrees to have Syntocinon?

Scenario 2

Judith is attending antenatal clinic; she is now 40 weeks pregnant with no signs of labour. She asks her midwife if she has any suggestions that might help labour get started. She has heard that eating a really hot curry might do the trick, but she does not think she could cope with the heartburn it would precipitate.

Practice point

Further research is needed to explore the effectiveness of some of the 'old wives' tales' that circulate regarding getting labour started. There is conclusive evidence that 'stretch and sweep' results in fewer inductions for post-maturity and this should be offered following discussion of the side-effects and benefits.

Further questions specific to Scenario 2 include:

1. What information has Judith received regarding the span of a normal pregnancy and the risks associated with post-maturity?
2. What evidence is there to support the use of nipple stimulation as a means of inducing labour?
3. Is there any evidence examining the use of hot baths, enemas and castor oil as methods of inducing labour?

4. Are there any contraindications to 'stretch and sweep' of the membranes?
5. Are there any herbal supplements that proclaim to help labour become established?
6. Is membrane sweeping acceptable to women as a method of ripening the cervix?

Conclusion

The issue of induction and acceleration of labour is fraught with debate and complicated by a range of potential courses of action. Despite evidence-based guidance, practice continues to vary between maternity units. Women undergoing such intervention require information about how their labour is progressing and what might happen next. Caring for women experiencing induction and augmentation of labour provides an excellent opportunity to develop a lasting relationship with a woman and her partner, providing continuous and individualized support.

Resources

Association of Radical Midwives: Induction: http://www.radmid.demon. co.uk/induction.htm.

Home birth organization: VBAC and induction or acceleration of labour: http://www.homebirth.org.uk/ vbacinduction.htm.

Patient UK Active management and induction: http://www.radmid.demon. co.uk/induction.htm.

Women's Health Information: Induction: http://www.womens-health. co.uk/induction.asp.

References

Areskog B, Uddenberg N, Kjessler B: Postnatal emotional balance in women with and without antenatal fear of childbirth, *Journal of Psychosomatic Research* 28:213–220, 1984.

Beigi A, Kabiri M, Zarrinkoub F: Cervical ripening with oral misoprostol at term, *International Journal of Gynaecology and Obstetrics* 83:251–255, 2003.

Bishop E: Pelvic scoring for elective induction, *Obstetrics and Gynecology* 24:267, 1964.

Boulvain M, Kelly A, Lohse C, et al: Mechanical methods for induction of labour DOI: 10.1002/14651858.CD001233, *Cochrane Database of Systematic Reviews* 4(CD001233), 2001.

Boulvain M, Stan C, Irion O: Membrane sweeping for induction of labour DOI: 10.1002/14651858.CD000451.pub2, *Cochrane Database of Systematic Reviews* 4(CD000451), 2004.

Bricker L, Lukas M: Amniotomy alone for induction of labour DOI: 10.1002/14651858.CD002862, *Cochrane Database of Systematic Reviews* 4(CD002862), 2000.

Chamberlain G, Zander L: ABC of labour care, *Induction. British Medical Journal,* 318:995–998, 1999.

D'Aniello G, Bocchi C, Florio P, et al: Cervical ripening and induction of labor by prostaglandin E2: a comparison between intracervical gel and vaginal pessary, *Journal of Maternal, Fetal and Neonatal Medicine* 14(3):158–162, 2003.

Department of Health: *Safety first: a report for patients, clinicians and healthcare managers,* London, 2006, Department of Health.

Fisher S, Mackenzie V, Davies G: Oral versus vaginal misoprostol for induction of labour: a double-blind randomised controlled trial, *American Journal of Obstetrics & Gynecology* 185:906–910, 2001.

Goeree R, Hannah M, Hewson S: Cost-effectiveness of induction of labour versus serial antenatal monitoring in the Canadian Multicentre Post-term Pregnancy Trial, *Canadian Medical Association Journal* 152:1445–1450, 1995.

Goldberg A, Wing D: Induction of labour: the misoprostol controversy, *Journal of Midwifery and Women's Health* 48(4):244–248, 2003.

Gülmezoglu AM, Crowther CA, Middleton P: Induction of labour for improving birth outcomes for women at or beyond term DOI: 10.1002/14651858.CD004945.pub2, *Cochrane Database of Systematic Reviews* 4(CD004945), 2006.

Heffner L, Elkin E, Fretts R: Impact of labor induction, gestational age, and maternal age on cesarean delivery rates, *Obstetrics and Gynecology* 102(2):287–293, 2003.

Heimstad R, Skogvoll E, Matteson L, et al: Induction of labour or serial antenatal fetal monitoring in postterm pregnancy: a randomized controlled trial, *Obstetrics and Gynecology* 109(3):609–617, 2007.

Hilder L, Costeloe K, Thilaganathan B: Prolonged pregnancy: evaluating gestation-specific risks of fetal and infant mortality, *British Journal of Obstetrics and Gynaecology* 105(2):169–173, 1998.

Hodnett E, Hannah M, Weston J, et al: Women's evaluations of induction of labor versus expectant management for prelabor rupture of the membranes at term. TermPROM Study Group, *Birth* 24(4):212–214, 1997.

Hofmeyr G, Gülmezoglu A: Vaginal misoprostol for cervical ripening and induction of labour, *Cochrane Database of Systematic Reviews* 1(CD000941), 2003.

Howarth GR, Botha DJ: Amniotomy plus intravenous oxytocin for induction of labour DOI: 10.1002/14651858. CD003250, *Cochrane Database of Systematic Reviews* 3(CD003250), 2001.

Johnson R, Taylor W: *Skills for midwifery practice*, ed 2, Edinburgh, 2006, Elsevier.

Kelly AJ, Kavanagh J, Thomas J: *Vaginal prostaglandin (PGE2 and PGF2a) for induction of labour at term (Cochrane Review)* The Cochrane Library 4, Chichester, UK, 2003, John Wiley.

Lieberman E, O'Donoghue C: Unintended effects of epidural analgesia during labour: a systematic review, *American Journal of Obstetrics and Gynecology* 186(5):s31–s68, 2002.

Mozurkewich E, Horrocks J, Daley S, et al: The MisoPROM study: a multicenter randomized comparison of oral misoprostol and oxytocin for premature rupture of membranes at term, *American Journal of Obstetrics & Gynecology* 189(4):1026–1030, 2003.

Neilson JP: Mifepristone for induction of labour DOI: 10.1002/14651858. CD002865, *Cochrane Database of Systematic Reviews* 4(CD002865), 2000.

National Institute for Health and Clinical Excellence (NICE): *Induction of labour. Inherited clinical guideline D*, London, 2001, NICE.

National Institute for Health and Clinical Excellence (NICE): *Intrapartum care. Care of healthy women and their babies during childbirth. NICE Clinical Guideline 55*, London, 2007, NICE.

National Institute for Health and Clinical Excellence (NICE): *Induction of labour*, London, 2008, NICE.

Sims E, Newman R, Hulsey T: Vaginal birth after cesarean: to induce or not to induce, *American Journal of Obstetrics & Gynecology* 184(6):1122–1124, 2001.

The Information Centre: NHS Maternity Statistics, England: 2005–2006, 2007. Online. Available http://www.ic.nhs.uk/webfiles/ publications/maternity0506/ NHSMaternityStatsEngland200506_ fullpublication%20V3.pdf December 11, 2008.

Williams F, Florey C, Ogston S, et al: UK study of intrapartum care for low risk primigravids: a survey of interventions, *Journal of Epidemiology and Community Health* 52(8):494–500, 1998.

Chapter 8

The second stage of labour

Trigger scenario

Lucy was about to birth her third baby. She suddenly had the urge to push, and the vertex was visible and advancing. The midwife was calmly preparing for the birth and putting her gloves on when another contraction started. The student could see that the midwife was not quite ready, and said to Lucy, 'Try not to push.' The midwife said, 'No, it's fine; you push if you need to.'

Introduction

The second stage of labour starts when the cervix is fully dilated, and ends when the baby is born. For some women (especially for multigravidae), this stage is relatively short; for others, it is prolonged and seems to last forever. The student midwife needs to learn how to recognize when labour is progressing effectively. This

chapter describes issues regarding the care the midwife provides during the second stage. Some women need assistance to give birth to their baby, and the indications and procedure for episiotomy, forceps and ventouse will be described. Issues surrounding the third stage of labour and perineal repair will be discussed in Chapters 9 and 11 respectively.

Recognizing the second stage

As each labour progresses at its own unique pace – depending on the position of the baby, parity, length, strength and frequency of contraction – recognizing when the transition from first stage to second stage has been reached is an essential midwifery skill. Being able to identify that a woman is in second stage when you greet her at the labour ward doors will dictate your next actions, and make a difference to her overall experience.

The signs that second stage is being approached or has been reached include: presenting part becomes visible, anus dilates, woman wishes to push with contractions and may do so involuntarily, and/or the vulva becomes congested. With experience, the student midwife will also recognize changes in the woman's behaviour, her voice and posture. Uterine contractions become less frequent but last longer. Hobbs (1998) describes how cervical dilatation can be estimated by observing the progression of a thin purple line up the natal cleft towards the sacral dimple at full dilatation. It may not be necessary to confirm full dilatation of the cervix by vaginal examination (VE) if the woman has been making good progress, continues to have regular strong contractions, does not have an epidural and the presenting part is visible at the introitus. However, if there has been delay during first stage of labour, and there was any evidence of caput succedaneum at previous VEs, then full dilatation should be confirmed. It is important to feel gently all the way around the presenting part as, occasionally, a rim or lip or cervix can be reluctant to dilate.

If the woman has an epidural in situ, and external signs suggest that full dilatation may have been reached, assessment will depend on how the epidural is being managed and on current local policy. If the epidural is not continuous but is being managed by top-ups, then full dilatation should be confirmed via VE prior to administration of the next top-up. If full

dilatation has been reached, and there is no evidence of fetal compromise, a further top-up may be administered to enable further descent of the fetal head. Alternatively, it may have been agreed with the woman that the epidural should be allowed to wear off to enable her to feel her contractions and respond to them. However, suddenly to experience second-stage contractions after being pain-free can be difficult to cope with, and the woman will need a lot of support to adjust to the pain.

Care during the second stage

Immediate vs delayed pushing

The evidence on immediate pushing versus delayed pushing is contradictory. A randomized controlled trial (RCT) of primigravidae with continuous epidural analgesia (Fitzpatrick et al 2002) did not find any difference regarding mode of birth between those who began pushing as soon as second stage was confirmed and those who waited an hour. Another study of primigravidae with continuous epidurals (Plunkett et al 2003) compared duration of pushing in second stage in those who pushed immediately and those who waited for an urge to push. They found no difference between the groups for duration of pushing or rates of spontaneous vaginal birth. However, a multi-centre RCT of delayed pushing for primigravidae with continuous epidural found that spontaneous birth was more frequent among women in the delayed pushing group (delay of 2 hours or more) (Fraser et al 2000).

Passive second stage of labour

Passive second stage of labour is defined as:

'the finding of full dilatation of the cervix prior to or in the absence of involuntary expulsive contractions'

(NICE 2007:29).

Although it may be confirmed that the cervix is fully dilated, while the presenting part remains high the woman may not have an urge to push. Subsequent contractions will cause the fetus to advance and stretch the soft tissues of the vagina. Further advancement will lead to stretching of the pelvic floor fascia, and exert pressure on the rectum combined with an associated urge to bear down. Although most women without an epidural experience an overwhelming urge to push, some do not (McKay et al 1990). A meta-analysis of the research comparing immediate versus passive descent in women with an epidural concluded that when passive descent is practised the risk of birth complications is reduced (Brancato et al 2008). The student midwife will gain valuable experience observing the range of women's responses to second stage of labour. S/he will learn to judge when to provide guidance and when to follow the woman's lead.

Active second stage of labour

Active second stage of labour is defined as:

- The presenting part is visible
- Expulsive contractions with a finding of full dilatation of the cervix or other sign of full dilatation of the cervix
- Active maternal effort following confirmation of full dilatation of the cervix in the absence of expulsive contractions.

During the active phase of the second stage of labour, the woman is pushing with contractions. This requires a lot of effort on her part, especially for the primigravida. She may become very hot from her exertions and will be grateful for sips of iced water and a gentle face wash with a familiar facecloth. These tasks can be undertaken by her partner, helping him/her to feel a valuable part of the birthing team. The woman may become frustrated at times, feeling that her efforts are not achieving any progress. She may behave out of character, perhaps by swearing or lashing out. However, joking with her partner about her behaviour should be avoided as this can undermine the trust she has placed in your loyalty and respect. It would be more appropriate to update her on her progress, reassure her that the baby is fine and praise her stamina.

Positions for second stage

Women should be encouraged to adopt the most comfortable position for them.

The position adopted for a labour that is progressing normally should be to the advantage of the woman rather than of her attendant. Although it can be challenging to a midwife for a woman to give birth in a position other than semi-recumbent on the bed, the benefits to the woman of being active during the birth are significant. In a systematic review of the evidence relating to alternative positions during second stage, Gupta & Hofmeyr (2004) concluded that pushing is more effective when an upright posture is adopted, and is associated with shorter duration of second stage, fewer episiotomies and assisted births. Upright positions can reduce the likelihood of vena-caval compression impeding fetal oxygenation. If progress has slowed down, a change in position can help fetal descent.

Activity

Identify five alternative positions for birth.

Consider why an upright position is associated with less obstetric intervention.

Find out what facilities there are in the unit where you work to facilitate 'off-the-bed' birth.

Directed or undirected pushing

Traditionally, women have been encouraged to take a deep breath, put their chin on their chest and push for up to 30 seconds (Valsalva manoeuvre). However, this technique leads to reduced blood flow to the uterus and lower cord blood pH (Enkin et al 2000). Women who are left to find their own pattern of pushing usually employ a combination of techniques, including pushing accompanied by the release of air. In the absence of fetal compromise, women should be encouraged to push as they feel the need (NICE 2007). In a randomized study comparing spontaneous pushing and the Valsalva technique, the babies in the spontaneous group had higher Apgar scores and umbilical cord pH and PO_2 levels and the women felt that they pushed more effectively than women in the Valsalva group (Yildirim & Beji 2008). However, women who have an epidural in situ may need some assistance in developing an effective pushing technique. Much encouragement is necessary; sometimes the use of a mirror, so that the woman can see the presenting part advancing, provides useful feedback.

Monitoring maternal and fetal wellbeing

At the onset of the active phase of the second stage, baseline observations of maternal temperature, pulse and blood pressure should be recorded on the partogram. The woman should be encouraged to pass urine to avoid trauma to an over-distended bladder. The time at which active pushing starts should be noted, along with the length, strength and frequency of contractions.

Details of progress should be documented half-hourly on the partogram, and include an assessment of how the women is coping with this strenuous activity. Maternal pulse and blood pressure should be repeated hourly, temperature continued 4-hourly (NICE 2007).

The colour of the liquor is noted as it drains onto a frequently replaced sanitary towel. When women are low risk and making good progress, the fetal heart should be auscultated after a contraction (for at least 60 seconds) at least every 5 minutes during the active phase of labour (NICE 2007) using a pinnard or fetal Doppler. If the fetal heart appears to deviate from the normal 110–160 beats per minute, the maternal pulse should be checked to differetiate the two (NICE 2007). Ideally, all documentation should be completed at the woman's side; this should not prevent supportive interaction.

Preparing for the birth

Confirmation of the second stage of labour does not mean 'panic'. It requires the midwife to prepare calmly and quietly for the imminent birth, while continuing to care for the woman and her partner. Generally, the midwife has more time to prepare when caring for a primigravida. However, the unique nature of childbirth means that slow progress cannot be assumed. The woman should not be left alone during the second stage. It is important that the midwife who is coordinating the labour suite is aware that the woman

has progressed to this stage. The woman should be introduced to an identified second midwife (where this practice is unit policy). This midwife will focus her care on the newborn baby while the first midwife continues to care for the woman. In some units, only one midwife is present for the birth, with practical assistance from another healthcare worker. However, another midwife should always be available, hence the need for two midwives at a home birth.

The midwife must ensure that all equipment that might be needed is in working order and available for use. The room should be warm, with no overpowering lights or other distractions. Interruptions should be kept to a minimum; the woman should feel that her room is private and secure. She may wish to play some music during the birth. Her wishes should be accommodated wherever possible.

Activity

Consider what preparations the midwife will make for the baby.
Think about how the room can be personalized for the birth.

As the presenting part advances with contractions, it will initially recede in between. This is normal as the perineal muscles are stretched and thinned. Progressively, a little more of the fetal head will become visible, and the partner can provide feedback to the woman about the amount of hair that can be seen. The midwife can now begin to prepare for the baby's arrival by making ready her equipment and creating a sterile field. This sterile field can be created anywhere – for example, on a tray on the floor – to suit the woman's chosen position and place of birth. However, the general concept of knowing where equipment can quickly be brought to hand, while not increasing the woman's risk of acquiring infection, should be maintained yet flexibly practised. The vulva and perineum should be swabbed with warm water, and a sterile pad placed over the anus. Cord clamps should be placed in the foreground of the field, with the scissors for cord-cutting and episiotomy at arm's length. Care should be taken not to contaminate your sterile gloves.

A rapidly advancing fetal head may mean that the delivery pack is being opened while you quickly put on sterile gloves, but the woman must remain your focus rather than a beautifully arranged sterile field. She should not be prevented from pushing, but you will need to gain eye contact with her and gently encourage her to listen to your voice. Before the next contraction you can coach her in what you will be asking her to do during the birth of the head. Ask her to blow out gently as the head crowns. This slow birth of the head will minimize the trauma to the perineum.

Minimizing perineal trauma

Woman-focused care

Probably one of the most important factors in helping the woman to minimize trauma to her perineum is through the development of a trusting relationship. It is crucial to develop a dialogue with her so that she knows that you are involving her in decisions about her care. She will develop confidence in your skills, and value the suggestions you make. Expecting her to respond to shouting, 'Don't push!', when you have hardly spent any time with her is a tall order. She is much more likely to respond to your voice at the crucial moment of crowning if she has heard your encouraging words throughout her labour.

Perineal massage

Antenatal perineal massage has been shown to reduce the incidence of second- and third-degree tears and episiotomies (Beckmann & Garrett 2006), particularly in women aged 30 or above (Shipman et al 1997). In an observational study of the acceptability of perineal massage (Labrecque et al 2001), women from 34–35 weeks' gestation were advised to undertake 5 to 10 minutes' daily massaging of the perineum. The study concluded that this practice was seen positively by women, and that most said they would do it in a subsequent pregnancy and recommend it to other pregnant women. There is no evidence to support the use of perineal massage by health professionals during the second stage of labour (NICE 2007).

Guarding the perineum

Women experience a range of practices during the second stage of labour, with the aim of protecting the perineum from undue damage and assisting the birth of the shoulders. The HOOP trial (Hands On Or Poised) was designed to compare two methods of perineal management during the second stage of labour (McCandlish et al 1998). 'Hands on' required the midwife to use one hand to flex the fetal head and the other to support or 'guard' the perineum – birth of the shoulders was assisted by lateral flexion. 'Hands poised' required the midwife to allow spontaneous birth of the head and shoulders, without touching the perineum.

The primary outcome for the trial was postpartum pain. There were significant differences between the two groups regarding perineal pain reported by women at 10 days postpartum, with more women in the 'hands poised' group reporting pain in the previous 24 hours. However, women in this group were less likely to have an episiotomy but more likely to require a manual removal of the placenta. The results of this trial provide valuable information for midwives when discussing second-stage management with women.

Episiotomy

An episiotomy is a surgical incision made in the perineum to facilitate birth of the presenting part of the fetus. Although once routine, systematic review of the evidence confirms that this practice should be restricted to clinical need (Renfrew et al 1998) and should not form part of routine care during spontaneous birth (NICE 2007).

Indications for episiotomy include fetal heart rate anomolies and maternal exhaustion or distress, and when the perineum is preventing adequate progress. When the midwife considers that episiotomy is required, she must inform the woman of her rationale in language that she can easily comprehend; verbal consent must be gained prior to the procedure (see Box 8.1) and following administration of local anaesthetic (Fig. 8.1). It should be performed only when the presenting part has descended onto the perineum, to allow the levator ani muscle to have been laterally displaced. The technique of preference is a mediolateral incision starting at the fourchette and directed to the right side (NICE 2007) (Fig. 8.2).

Nuchal cord

Following the birth of the head, it is common practice in the UK for midwives to run their index finger under the baby's occiput towards the nape of the neck, which is still in the vagina (Downe 2004). This is to establish whether or not the umbilical cord is around the baby's neck (nuchal cord), potentially impeding the flow of blood to the brain. A small study examining the practice of detecting nuchal cord antenatally through Doppler sonography (Aksoy 2003) found an incidence of 28% nuchal cord at birth. A randomized study did not find any adverse effects of cord entaglement (Sadan et al 2007). A loose cord could be looped over the baby's head prior to birth of the body so that it cannot tighten during the birth. Alternatively, a tight cord could be

Box 8.1 Procedure for episiotomy

• Inform the woman of the situation that you feel warrants the need for an episiotomy

Rationale So that the woman can make a judgment about the situation and be fully involved in her care

• Gain verbal consent from the woman to perform an episiotomy

Rationale This is a surgical procedure and requires informed consent

• Ask assistant to open 10 ml syringe and needle onto sterile field

Rationale In preparation for administration of local anaesthetic

• Apply needle to the syringe, and withdraw plunger (if using local anaesthetic supplied in vial with rubber stopper)

Rationale In preparation for extracting local anaesthetic from glass vial

• Ask assistant to show you and check (drug, dosage, clear liquid and expiry date) local anaesthetic

Rationale To ensure correct drug has been selected and is in condition for safe administration

• While assistant holds vial upside down, position needle into centre of rubber bung and insert some air

Rationale To facilitate withdrawal of drug from a vacuumed vessel

• Withdraw 10 ml of 0.5% (or 5 ml of 1%) lignocaine, and check amount with assistant

Rationale To check that correct amount of drug has been prepared

• If right-handed, insert index and middle fingers of left hand in between the presenting part and the perineum, pointing downwards, and make perineal skin accessible

Rationale To protect the presenting part from the local anaesthetic

• In between contractions, insert needle into perineum along the line of the intended episiotomy site. Withdraw the plunger and, if no blood returns into the syringe, inject 2-3 ml. Repeat either side of the intended site (Fig. 8.1).

Rationale To anaesthetize the skin around the intended episiotomy avoiding a maternal vein

• Dispose of needle and syringe in appropriate sharps bin

Rationale To avoid needle stick injury to midwife, woman, baby or assistants

• If fetal and maternal conditions allow, wait for two contractions

Rationale To allow local anaesthetic to take effect

• If right-handed, insert index and middle fingers of left hand in between the presenting part and the perineum, pointing downwards

Rationale To protect the presenting part from the episiotomy scissors and make perineal skin accessible

• With right hand, take the open scissors and position in between presenting part and perineum, over area of intended episiotomy

Rationale To find optimum position in readiness for next uterine contraction

continued

Box 8.1 Continued

• At height of next contraction, and with maternal effort applying the presenting part on to the perineum, turn scissor blades at right angles to the skin and make single cut

Rationale   To aid thinning of perineum prior to incision, aiding performance of episiotomy and reducing blood loss

• Apply even pressure to the advancing presenting part with left hand. Inform woman of her progress

Rationale   To prevent uncontrolled expulsion of presenting part, which might result in further perineal trauma. To continue to involve the woman in her progress

• Reposition used episiotomy scissors at far end of sterile field, beyond the cord clamps

Rationale   To avoid mistaking episiotomy scissors for cord clamps

• Continue with the birth as normal

Rationale   To continue involving the woman in the birth of her baby

• Apply pressure to episiotomy site with sterile pad, if actively bleeding

Rationale   To minimize blood loss, awaiting suturing

• Document indications, consent, local anaesthetic, position and blood loss

Rationale   To comply with professional guidance

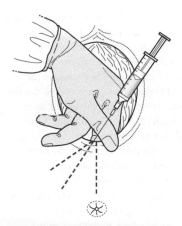

Fig. 8.1 Administering local anaesthetic in preparation for episiotomy. (From Johnson & Taylor 2006, with permission.)

clamped and cut, then unravelled prior to the birth.

However, the value of these practices has been contested (Wickham 2003) and they are seen as dangerous and invasive by some practitioners. To cut the cord of a baby who then has shoulder dystocia would run the risk of terminating its supply of oxygen for several minutes (Johnson & Taylor 2006), leading to potentially irreversible brain damage. Following a review of four cases where the physician had severed the nuchal cord prior to the birth of the body, Iffy et al (2001) concluded that it is a dangerous

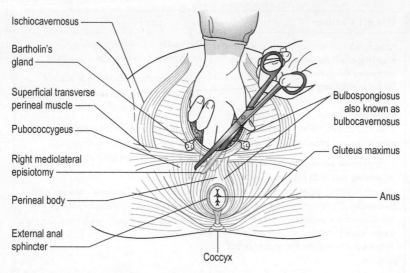

Ischiocavernosus

Bartholin's gland

Superficial transverse perineal muscle

Pubococcygeus

Right mediolateral episiotomy

Perineal body

External anal sphincter

Coccyx

Bulbospongiosus also known as bulbocavernosus

Gluteus maximus

Anus

Fig. 8.2 Diagram of an episiotomy showing the superficial muscles involved. (From Henderson & Macdonald 2004.)

procedure that should be avoided. Similarly, looping the cord over the baby's head is not without risk. Cases are described where the cord has snapped (Reed 2007) and handling the cord can precipitate spasm of the blood vessels impeding the baby's blood supply (Coad & Dunstall 2006). A random sample of American nurse-midwives (Mercer et al 2000) revealed that 96% of respondents avoided clamping a nuchal cord where possible. Jackson et al (2007) found that some midwives changed their practice in response to adverse incidents, towards less intervention. The NICE intrapartum care guidelines do not mention feeling for nuchal cord; further research and debate is required on this aspect of midwifery care.

Birth of the shoulders

Once the head is birthed and restitution and external rotation has occurred, the baby is positioned for birth of the shoulders. If the woman is semi-recumbent, the midwife cradles the head between her hands and guides the head down towards the bed or floor, to birth the anterior shoulder. When this has escaped under the symphysis pubis, the midwife guides the head upwards towards the woman to deliver the posterior shoulder. The woman can then assist with birth of the body if she wishes. Using this method prevents potentially both shoulders coming through the perineum at the same time and is useful for assisting women with an epidural in situ. However, some women prefer a hands-off approach, particulary if kneeling or standing, and these choices should be discussed before second stage (see HOOP Study, above).

Water birth

Second-stage management during a water birth is very much 'hands off' while the usual observations are recorded. In addition, water temperature and maternal temperature are taken regularly in accordance with local policy. When the baby is born, it should be brought straight to the surface of the water. Water birth should only be conducted or closely supervised by experienced midwives.

Particular care should be taken to note the condition of the umbilical cord following a water birth. Cro & Preston (2002) present a number of case histories of successful water births that were then complicated by snapping of the cord. This is a potentially dangerous situation, as the water is likely to be discoloured following birth – making it difficult to note a sudden change in its colour due to a ruptured cord. Care should be taken not to put undue traction on the cord as the baby is brought to the surface and to actively establish the condition of the cord following the birth.

Delay in the second stage of labour

To have successfully negotiated the first stage of labour, and then not be able to push the baby out, is particularly demoralizing. One study exploring risk factors for arrest of descent during second stage (Feinstein et al 2002) identified the following factors: nulliparity, macrosomia, epidural analgesia, hydramnios, hypertensive disorders, gestational diabetes, male gender, premature rupture of the membranes and induction of labour.

The NICE intrapartum care guidelines suggest that a vaginal examination is performed in response to the woman's request or hourly during the second stage of labour, preceded by abdominal palpation. A diagnosis of delay is made when the second stage has lasted 2 hours in a nulliparous woman and 1 hour in a parous woman (NICE 2007:29). They recommend that women should then be referred to an appropriate healthcare professional for an instrumental vaginal birth. Diagnosis of the underlying problem – for example, malposition – will be made before the appropriate action can be taken. All referrals should be documented, followed by an assessment of the clinical situation and a plan of action discussed and agreed with the woman.

Instrumental birth

There are two methods for assisting the vaginal birth of the fetus during second stage of labour: forceps delivery and ventouse (vacuum). Both require a skilled operator. A systematic review comparing vacuum extraction with forceps for assisted vaginal delivery (Johanson & Menon 1998) concluded that the vacuum reduces maternal morbidity but increases the incidence of retinal haemorrhages and cephalhaematoma in the neonate. Serious injury with either instrument is rare and the choice of instrument often depends on the experience of the operator (Royal College of Obstetricians & Gynaecologists (RCOG) 2005).

When the decision is made to birth the baby via forceps or ventouse, the woman and her partner will require detailed information about what is about to happen. Reassurance that you will stay with them is an important start. Working in a busy obstetric unit, such occurrences will become part of the student midwife's routine, but they can be frightening experiences for those on the receiving end. This fear can be minimized by maintaining a relaxed environment and by showing confidence in the practitioner who is about to birth the baby. Parents need to be warned that sterile packs will be opened and that equipment makes clattering noises as it is being placed on a metal trolley. They can be assured that, although there will be more people present at the birth, you will introduce any newcomer. A second midwife will come in (hopefully already introduced), and will check the resuscitaire. A paediatrician may be on hand, and will also check the resuscitaire.

Adequate analgesia must be assured prior to instrumental delivery. Forceps delivery in particular will be uncomfortable for a woman without an epidural in situ. If time does not permit insertion of an epidural, a pudendal nerve block may be administered by the doctor (RCOG 2005).

While most practitioners choose to have women in the lithotomy position when using forceps or ventouse, this is not always essential. Charles (2002) describes how birth can be achieved when two assistants gently hold the woman's heels. The partner should stay at the head of the bed to support the woman, and the midwife will palpate contractions. The vulva will be swabbed, and drapes arranged to create a sterile field. The operator will confirm the position of the fetus and position the forceps or ventouse. When the next contraction occurs, gentle traction will be applied to bring the head down onto the perineum while maternal effort is made. If forceps are being used, most operators will perform an episiotomy prior to birth of the head (Macleod & Murphy 2008). There is no evidence to suggest that prophylactic antibiotics reduce the risk of maternal infection following operative vaginal birth (Liabsuetrakul et al 2004).

Midwife instrumental birth

A midwifery ventouse practitioner (MVP) can provide an alternative perspective for ventouse delivery. Being experienced in the progress of the second stage of labour, they are able to assess the situation in context and not rush in with the instruments as soon as they are called. Charles (2002) describes the sense of achievement when, after being called to a birth, she is able to leave the room without resorting to suction.

In an evaluation of the MVP course at Bournemouth University, researchers concluded that midwives who had undertaken the programme became more confident in their practice in general (Alexander et al 2002). They did not appear to undertake this new aspect of their role at the expense of their previous role, and remained cautious about the need for intervention. Porter (2003) also describes how midwives who have extended their roles to include simple lift-out ventouse extractions have grown in confidence. Their practice is grounded in supporting normal birth but they are alert to deviation from this path and open to seeking medical advice when necessary.

As with most instrumental births, maternal effort is invaluable. By bringing the head gently down onto the perineum, women who have not had an epidural (and where there is no fetal compromise) can be encouraged to birth the baby themselves. This allows the perineum more time to stretch, with the possibility of avoiding episiotomy or a tear, but also enables the woman to remain in control. Wills & Deighton (2002) describe how women can still feel that they had a 'normal' birth even when there was some instrumental involvement.

Activity

List the potential advantages and disadvantages of midwives undertaking instrumental births.

Find out if there are any MVPs in the unit where you work. If so, find time to talk to them and ask them about some of the births they have assisted.

With baby

As the end of second stage approaches, the woman should again be asked if she wants the baby delivered directly onto her abdomen. For a woman giving birth on all fours or standing, the midwife can encourage her to take the baby up herself. Immediate contact with the baby should always be encouraged. If, however, she requests that the baby be dried off and cleaned up before she holds him/her, this activity can be undertaken by her side with a running commentary that directly involves her. For example, 'I'm just drying her head so that she doesn't get cold ... look how she is looking around her [to woman] ... look, here's your mum [to baby]', etc.

Robinson (2002) highlights how important it is to respect the fact that the baby belongs to the parents, not to the midwives. Consent should always be sought before anything is done to the baby, and within sight of the parents where possible. During an emergency this may not be possible or appropriate, but parents should be continually informed of what is happening.

If the woman wants to hold the baby straight away, then skin-to-skin contact should be offered, whether or not she intends to breastfeed. The mother can also actively participate in the drying ritual. Babies lose most heat from their heads, as this comprises a large proportion of the total body surface area. Heat loss is compounded by the fact that the baby is wet following the birth, hence the activity of drying the baby with a soft, warm towel. This towel should then be replaced with another warm, dry towel, continuing to keep the head covered, except during parental inspection of hair colour and seeing if the baby has his or her father's ears! Skin-to-skin contact has been shown to be the most effective way for maintaining a baby's body temperature and also correcting it in those who have become hypothermic (Christensson et al 1998). It supports effective transition to extrauterine life, including improved respiration and oxygen saturation (Ferber & Makhoul 2004).

In a prospective longitudinal study, Rowe-Murray & Fisher (2001) investigated the impact of mode of birth on women's emotional wellbeing and early contact with their baby. They found that the longer the time lapse between birth and holding the baby, the lower postpartum mood was. Length

of first contact did not contribute significantly to postpartum mood.

Activity

Think about how achievement of 'baby friendly' status would potentially impact on the postpartum mood of women who give birth there.

Make sure you understand why it is so important that the baby does not get cold following birth.

Reflection on trigger

Look back on the trigger scenario.

Lucy was about to birth her third baby. She suddenly had the urge to push, and the vertex was visible and advancing. The midwife was calmly preparing for the birth and putting her gloves on when another contraction started. The student could see that the midwife was not quite ready, and said to Lucy, 'Try not to push.' The midwife said, 'No, it's fine; you push if you need to.'

Now that you are familiar with the second stage of labour you should have insight into how the scenario relates to the evidence about it. The jigsaw model will now be used to explore the trigger scenario in more depth.

Effective communication

It is essential that the midwife and woman are communicating effectively throughout the second stage of labour to ensure that the woman remains motivated and focused. In order to listen carefully to the midwife's feedback about the progress of the advancing head, the woman needs to trust and value what she is saying. Questions that arise from the scenario might include: Why did the student ask the woman not to push? How did Lucy feel when the student midwife told her not to push? Could the midwife have re-phrased her response – if so, how? Had there been any discussion about listening to the midwife for information as the head was being born?

Woman-centred care

It is evident from the scenario that the midwife did not want to impose restrictions on the woman, by asking her not to push until the midwife was ready. She wanted the woman to go with the flow of what her body was doing naturally. Questions that arise from the scenario might include: Had the woman and midwife met previously? Had the midwife discussed with the woman what position she might like to be in for the birth? What antenatal processes support woman-centred care during the birth? How could the midwife have involved the woman further at this stage?

Using best evidence

The length of second stage varies considerably between individual women. There is also a range of evidence to support different midwifery

practices during this time of heightened anticipation. Questions that arise from the scenario might include: What factors influence the length of second stage in women? Which of those factors might have applied to this woman? What evidence is there to support the use of alternative positions for birth? Why was the student uncomfortable with the woman pushing before the midwife had her gloves on? What does the evidence say about the outcome if the midwife does not support the perineum as the head crowns?

Professional and legal issues

The midwife supporting Lucy was calm and confident. Questions that arise from the scenario might include: What factors contributed to the midwife's cool demeanour? How many births had the student midwife witnessed and why was it not she who was preparing for the birth? Is the European Union Directive that 'students should personally carry out at least 40 deliveries' (NMC 2004:34) appropriate? How could this directive be further enhanced? Which aspects of the Code (NMC 2008) are particularly pertinent to this scenario?

Team working

Many individuals contribute to the care of women in labour either directly, such as the midwife, or indirectly, such as the ward clerks and healthcare assistants. Questions that arise from the scenario might include: Had the student midwife worked with this midwife before? Why were the student and midwife not appearing to be working as a team and how could this have been avoided? How had the student's mentor facilitated the student's awareness of multi-disciplinary working? How many individual healthcare workers had contributed in some way to the care of this labouring woman?

Clinical dexterity

Student midwives observe a range of practices by midwives as they progress through their pre-registration programme. Questions that arise from the scenario might include: Why was the midwife not ready for the birth? What are the implications of helping a woman birth without wearing gloves? What are the implications of helping a woman birth without having the cord clamps ready? What are the priorities in terms of preparation, when a parous woman says she want to push? How many different ways have you observed midwives behave in preparation for a baby's arrival? How have these observations informed your current practice?

Models of care

Women give birth in a range of different environments, depending on the local models of care available to them. Questions that arise from the scenario might include: Was the woman at home or in a hospital labour ward? How might the environment have influenced the midwife's response to the student's

request? How might the environment have influenced how the woman responded to the student or midwife? How might the environment influence who was present for the birth? How might the models of care influence the midwife's job satisfaction and workload?

Safe environment

Women in labour need to feel safe and cared for by competent staff. The student and the midwife in the scenarios were giving mixed messages. Questions that arise from the scenario might include: How might the request 'Try not to push' be interpreted by the woman in terms of her safety at that time? What actions can the midwife take during the second stage of labour to help a woman feel safe? How can the midwife help the birthing partner feel safe at this time? How could the midwife have helped the student midwife feel safe?

Promotes health

There are many opportunities throughout the birthing process that midwives can utilize to promote health and wellbeing. Questions that arise from the scenario might include: Has the midwife discussed with the woman the benefits of her having skin-to-skin contact with the baby soon after birth? Has the midwife involved the father of the baby throughout the birth, to increase his confidence to interact with the baby when it is born? Has the woman partaken in any perineal massage during her pregnancy, to reduce the likelihood of sustaining perineal trauma at the birth?

Further scenarios

The following scenarios enable you to consider how specific situations influence the care the midwife provides. Use the jigsaw model to explore the issues raised in each scenario.

Scenario 1

Janette is in labour with her first baby. She has been actively pushing for over an hour. There has been some progress, but she is now very tired. 'I can't do this any more,' she sobs. 'Please get this baby out.'

Practice point

The second stage of labour can be very hard work, especially in nulliparous women. It is not uncommon for women who have experienced a long labour to lose faith in their body's ability to birth their baby. With appropriate support, however, the woman can find renewed energy and achieve a spontaneous birth. Sometimes, however, women need assistance, and the midwife must recognize when to refer her to an appropriate practitioner for an instrumental birth.

Further questions specific to Scenario 1 include:

1. What factors might be contributing to Janette's slow progress in the second stage of labour?

2. How can the midwife help Janette achieve a spontaneous vaginal birth?
3. What factors would alert the midwife that the woman might need an instrumental birth?
4. How can the midwife ensure that an instrumental birth is a positive experience?
5. What are the midwife's professional duties when referring a woman to another practitioner?

Scenario 2

Abigail is labouring at home in a pool with her partner James, anticipating the birth of their second baby. She appears to be progressing well and the midwife telephones her colleague to join them for the birth, which she feels will be in the next hour or so. As she finishes her conversation, Abigail has another contraction and begins pushing involuntarily. The midwife looks into the water to see the baby's head emerge.

Practice point

Labouring and giving birth in water is a choice that increasing numbers of women are exercising. Some midwives have had the opportunity to care for many women using water to help them relax in labour and have developed knowledge and expertise in supporting women with a pool birth. However, some midwives do not have such experience and need to develop their skills in this area in order to provide safe and competent care. Attendance at study days, in-house education and buddying with an experienced midwife are all useful sources of knowledge that can be accessed.

Further questions specific to Scenario 2 include:

1. How can midwives prepare to support a woman with a pool birth at home?

2. What action should the midwife take as she sees the baby's head emerge?

3. How can the environment be adapted to provide a safe place of birth?

4. What is James's role during the second stage of labour?

5. What is the impact of the water on the woman's perineum?

6. How would the midwife manage any delay during the second stage of labour in water?

7. Does the woman need to get out of the water for the third stage of labour?

Conclusion

Second stage of labour is a time of heightened anticipation for both the parents and the midwife. Recognizing effective progress during this phase of labour is a skill that all midwives must develop and fine-tune. The midwife must document this progress in a sequential, concise manner, remaining 'with woman' throughout.

Resources

Altman MR, Lydon-Rochelle MT: Prolonged second stage of labor and risk of adverse maternal and perinatal outcomes: a systematic review, *Birth* 33(4):315–322, 2006.

Association of Radical Midwives: positions for birth: http://www.radmid.demon.co.uk/position.htm.

Operative vaginal delivery, Royal College of Obstetricians and Gynaecologists: http://www.rcog.org.uk/resources/public/pdf/reentop26operativevaginaldelivery1207.pdf.

Patient UK: episiotomy and tears: http://www.patient.co.uk/showdoc/40000277.

Royal College of Midwives Virtual Institute: http://www.rcmnormalbirth.org.uk/webfiles/Related%20Articles/Reducing%20Interventions%2004.03.pdf.

Sampselle C, Miller J, Luecha Y, et al: Providing support of spontaneous pushing during the second stage of labour, *JOGN Nursing* 34: 695–702, 2005.

References

Aksoy U: Prenatal color Doppler sonographic evaluation of nuch encirclement by the umbilical cord, *Journal of Clinical Ultrasound* 31(9):473–477, 2003.

Alexander J, Anderson T, Cunningham S: An evaluation by focus group and survey of a course for Midwifery Ventouse Practitioners, *Midwifery* 18(2):165–172, 2002.

Beckmann M, Garrett A: Antenatal perineal massage for reducing perineal trauma, *Cochrane Database of Systematic Reviews*(CD005123), 2006.

Brancato R, Church S, Stone P: A meta-analysis of passive descent versus immediate pushing in nulliparous women with epidural analgesia in the second stage of labour, *JOGN Nursing* 37:4–12, 2008.

Charles C: Practising as a Midwife Ventouse Practitioner in an isolated midwife-led unit setting, *MIDIRS Midwifery Digest* 12(1):75–77, 2002.

Christensson K, Bhat G, Amadi B, et al: Randomised study of skin to skin versus incubator care for rewarming low-risk hypothermic neonates, *Lancet* 352(9134):1115, 1998.

Coad J, Dunstall M: *Anatomy and physiology for midwives*, ed 2, Edinburgh, 2006, Mosby.

Cro S, Preston J: Cord snapping at waterbirth delivery, *British Journal of Midwifery* 10(8):494–497, 2002.

Downe S: Care in the second stage of labour. In *Maye's midwifery. A text book for midwives*, Edinburgh, 2004, Baillière Tindall.

Enkin M, Keirse M, Neilson J, et al: *A guide to effective care in pregnancy and childbirth*, ed 3, Oxford, 2000, Oxford University Press.

Feinstein U, Sheiner E, Levy A, et al: Risk factors for arrest of descent during the second stage of labor, *International Journal of Gynecology and Obstetrics* 77(1):7–14, 2002.

Ferber S, Makhoul I: The effect of skin to skin contact (kangaroo care) shortly after birth on the neurobehavioural responses of the term newborn: a randomized, controlled trial, *Pediatrics* 113(4):858–865, 2004.

Fitzpatrick M, Harkin R, McQuillan K, et al: A randomised clinical trial comparing the effects of delayed versus immediate pushing with epidural analgesia on mode of delivery and faecal continence, *BJOG: An International Journal of Obstetrics and Gynaecology* 109(12):1359–1365, 2002.

Fraser W, Marcoux S, Krauss I, et al: Multicenter, randomised, controlled trial of delayed pushing for nulliparous women in the second stage of labour with continuous epidural analgesia. The PEOPLE (Pushing Early or Pushing Late with Epidural) Study Group, *American Journal of Obstetrics and Gynecology* 182(5):1165–1172, 2000.

Gupta J, Hofmeyr G: Position for women during second stage of labour. (Cochrane Review). In *The Cochrane Library, Issue 1*, Chichester, 2004, John Wiley.

Henderson C, Macdonald S (eds): *Mayes midwifery. A text book for midwives*, Edinburgh, 2004, Ballière Tindall.

Hobbs L: Assessing cervical dilatation without VEs: watching the purple line, *The Practising Midwife* 1(11):34–35, 1998.

Iffy L, Varadi V, Papp E: Untoward neonatal sequelae deriving from cutting of the umbilical cord before delivery, *Medical Law* 20(4):627–634, 2001.

Jackson H, Melvin C, Downe S: Midwives and the fetal nuchal cord: a survey of practices and perceptions, *Journal of Midwifery and Women's Health* 52(1):49–55, 2007.

Johanson R, Menon V: Vacuum extraction versus forceps for assisted vaginal delivery (Cochrane Review). In: *The Cochrane Library*, 1998. 4(10.1002/14651858). CD000224.

Johnson R, Taylor W: *Skills for midwifery practice*, ed 2, Edinburgh, 2006, Elsevier.

Labrecque M, Eason E, Marcoux S: Women's views on the practice of prenatal perineal massage, *British Journal of Obstetrics and Gynaecology* 108:499–504, 2001.

Liabsuetrakul T, Choobun T, Peeyananjarassri K, et al: Antibiotic prophylaxis for operative vaginal delivery DOI: 10.1002/14651858. CD004455.pub2, *Cochrane Database of Systematic Reviews* 3(CD004455), 2004.

Macleod M, Murphy D: Operative vaginal delivery and the use of episiotomy: a survey of practice in the United Kingdom and Ireland, *European Journal of Obstetrics & Gynecology and Reproductive Biology* 136(2):178–183, 2008.

McCandlish R, Bowler U, van Asten H, et al: A randomised controlled trial of care of the perineum during second stage of normal labour, *British Journal of Obstetrics and Gynaecology* 105(12):1262–1272, 1998.

McKay S, Barrows T, Roberts J: Women's views of second-stage labor as assessed by interviews and video tapes, *Birth* 17(4):192–198, 1990.

Mercer J, Nelson C, Skovgaard R: Umbilical cord clamping: beliefs and practices of American nurse-midwives, *Journal of Midwifery and Women's Health* 45(1):58–66, 2000.

National Institute for Health and Clinical Excellence (NICE): *Intrapartum care. Care of healthy women and their babies during childbirth. NICE clinical guideline 55*, London, 2007, NICE.

Nursing and Midwifery Council (NMC): *Standards of proficiency for pre-registration midwifery education*, London, 2004, NMC.

Nursing and Midwifery Council (NMC): *The Code. Standards of conduct, performance and ethics for nurse and midwives*, London, 2008, NMC.

Plunkett BA, Lin A, Wong CA, et al: Management of the second stage of labor in nulliparas with continuous epidural analgesia, *Obstetrics & Gynecology* 102(1):109–114, 2003.

Porter R: Expectations of the midwife's role: supporting normal birth, *MIDIRS Midwifery Digest* 13(2):217–219, 2003.

Reed R: Nuchal cords: think before you check, *The Practising Midwife* 10(5):18–20, 2007.

Renfrew MJ, Hannah W, Albers L, et al: Practices that minimize trauma to the genital tract in childbirth: a systematic review of the literature, *Birth* 25(3):143–160, 1998.

Robinson J: Separation from the baby – a cause of PTSD?, *British Journal of Midwifery* 10(9):548, 2002.

Rowe-Murray HJ, Fisher JRW: Operative intervention in delivery is associated with compromised early mother–infant interaction, *British Journal of Obstetrics and Gynaecology* 108(10):1068–1075, 2001.

Royal College of Obstetricians and Gynaecologists: Operative vaginal delivery. Green top guideline No 26, 2005. Online. Available http://www. rcog.org.uk/resources/Public/pdf/ greentop26OperativeVaginalDelivery 1207.pdf. December 11, 2008

Sadan O, Fleischfarb Z, Everon S, et al: Cord around the neck: should it be severed at delivery? A RCT, *American Journal of Perinatology* 25(1):61–64, 2007.

Shipman M, Boniface D, Tefft M, et al: Antenatal perineal massage and subsequent perineal outcomes: a andomised controlled trial, *British Journal of Obstetrics and Gynaecology* 104(7): 787–791, 1997.

Wickham S: To feel, or not to feel? Checking the nuchal cord, *The Practising Midwife* 6(2):27, 2003.

Wills J, Deighton S: Midwives performing instrumental deliveries. Programme development and personal reflection, *The Practising Midwife* 5(7): 22–25, 2002.

Yildirim G, Beji N: Effects of pushing techniques in birth on mother and fetus: a randomised study, *Birth* 35(1):25–30, 2008.

Chapter 9

The third stage of labour

Trigger scenario

The midwife wiped Liz's face with a cool flannel. 'Did you want to push with that contraction?' she asked. Liz kept her eyes closed and nodded. The gas and air was just wearing off. 'We'd better get ready then,' the midwife said. She turned to the student, 'Just check this Syntometrine for me.' Turning to the woman, she said, 'Are you happy to have the injection in your leg for the afterbirth?' But Liz was using the gas and air. Another contraction had started.

Introduction

Sometimes the art and science of midwifery combine to confuse and frustrate the novice midwife trying to get to grips with how things should be done. A student might think that there must surely be a 'best way' to manage a particular situation, so why don't all midwives practise in the same manner? Individual midwifery practice is influenced by many factors, including personal philosophy, previous experience, mentorship, delivery suite culture and, of course, hospital and national guidelines. Practice should be adapted to meet the needs of each woman who is cared for. Management of the third stage is one aspect of midwifery that is open to differing practice. This chapter aims to present the different perspectives, explore the evidence and outline safe practice.

Definition: third stage of labour

This is the interval from the birth of the baby to the complete expulsion of the placenta and membranes (NICE 2007). The process can be seen schematically in Fig. 9.1. Large studies (Combs & Laros 1991, Dombrowski et al 1995) have shown that as the length of third stage increases, particularly if it exceeds 30 minutes, the risk of postpartum

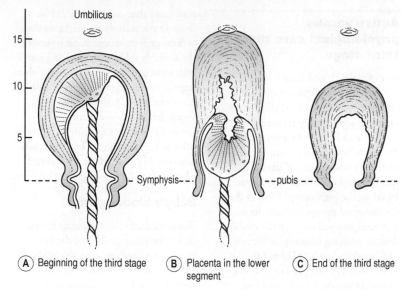

Fig. 9.1 Position of the uterus before and after placental separation. (From Johnson & Taylor 2006, with permission.)

haemorrhage (PPH) also rises. It follows that by reducing the length of the third stage, the amount of blood loss associated with this stage of labour is reduced. Thus, most labour wards employ a policy that requires midwives to manage actively the third stage of labour. The length of this period is accurately timed and documented in the woman's notes.

Activity

Outline the process by which the placenta separates from the uterine wall.

List three complications of third stage and how these can be minimized.

Find out what is meant by 'living ligature'.

Terminology

Active management of third stage in the UK involves the administration of an oxytocic drug to the woman after the birth of the baby's shoulder (to ensure that shoulder dystocia is not a possibility). The cord is clamped and cut when the baby is born. The placenta is delivered by controlled cord traction (CCT).

Physiological (natural or expectant) third-stage care requires the attendant to be patient and wait for the woman's body to do what it was designed to do. No oxytocics are given and the cord is not cut until either it stops pulsating or until after the placenta is expelled. The placenta is expelled by maternal effort.

Active versus physiological care during third stage

In 1988, the Bristol third stage trial (Prendiville et al 1988) reported that active management of the third stage of labour significantly reduced the incidence of PPH. It had set out to determine whether the routine policy of active management of labour was justified, and concluded that it was, based on the high rate of PPH in the physiological group. Indeed, the study had been stopped early by the trial's data monitoring committee because early analysis had highlighted the PPH issue. Despite the fact that the midwives involved in the trial had received training in the physiological management of third stage, this had not been their customary practice and thus was one of the study's weaknesses. They concluded that a randomized controlled trial should be conducted in a setting in which physiological management was the norm.

The views of women and midwives who took part in the Bristol trial were also collated and analysed (Harding et al 1989). The authors concluded that their views concurred with the findings from the main trial, and that active management was generally favoured above expectant care.

Another large trial was subsequently undertaken at Hinchingbrooke Hospital in Cambridgeshire, where midwives were already familiar with both active and expectant management of third stage (Rogers et al 1998). Again, it was concluded that the rate of PPH was lower in the actively managed women.

Subsequently, a systematic review of the available evidence comparing active with expectant management of the third stage of labour (Prendiville et al 2000:02) concluded that, 'Active management should be the routine management of choice for women expecting to deliver a baby by vaginal delivery in a maternity hospital.' However, there are potential advantages to a physiological third stage.

Baby's blood volume

When nature is left to take its course, no oxytocics are given and the cord continues to pulsate after the birth, the baby continues to receive blood from the placenta. Indeed, babies in the physiological group of the Bristol trial (Prendiville et al 1988) were on average 85 g heavier than those in the active management group, having received more blood than babies in the active group. A higher mean birthweight was also a finding of the Hinchingbrooke trial (Rogers et al 1998).

If the cord is clamped and cut as part of active management, then the baby is not receiving its quota of blood. This could be particularly problematic for the premature baby. In a randomized trial involving 36 premature babies born vaginally (Kinmond et al 1993), a practice of lowering the baby 20 cm below the level of the introitus for 30 seconds before the cord was clamped significantly increased the initial mean packed cell volume. None of the babies in the experimental group required a red cell transfusion. In a systematic review of the research regarding the timing of umbilical cord clamping (McDonald & Middleton 2008) it was concluded that delay of 2 to 3 minutes did not increase the risk of postpartum haemorrhage but did result in a raised iron status in the baby for up to 6 months and an increased risk of jaundice requiring phototherapy.

Informed choice?

Unfortunately, many women only become involved in a discussion about the third stage if they have requested the natural method. Of course, all midwives must gain verbal consent before giving an oxytocic, but the explanation and limited discussion often take place during labour – and this is inappropriate. An opportunity to discuss such interventions should take place antenatally, ideally in the woman's own home with a midwife she knows. The completion of the birth plan in the National Maternity Records or locally created document can facilitate this discussion. However, women only have a real choice if their attendants are confident and willing to provide either option. Anderson (1999:11) argues

that, following discussion about the relative advantages and disadvantages of both methods, 'women should then be supported in their choice by midwives skilled in both approaches to third stage care.' Although the NICE intrapartum care guidelines recommend active management, they also state that women at low risk of PPH who request physiological management should be 'supported in their choice' (NICE 2007:34). For a summary of management of third stage see Box 9.1.

For some women, part of the mystery of giving birth is learning about how their bodies respond to the demands of labour and birth. They may have endeavoured to go without drugs, either to ease or speed up their labour, and would also like to do the same for third stage. Having a physiological third stage when so many women have active management can be a valuable achievement. Many women in the physiological arm of the Hinchingbrooke trial (Rogers & Wood 1999) found satisfaction in the fact that they had birthed their babies without any intervention. Alternatively, it could be the redeeming factor of an otherwise difficult experience where previous choices had to be abandoned – for example, if transferred to hospital when a home birth had been planned.

Active management

Drugs used for active management

The preparation commonly administered is 1 ml Syntometrine, which includes

---

Box 9.1 Summary of the management of third stage

All women

- Antenatal discussion
- Wishes recorded in birth plan
- Review of birth plan in early labour

Physiological management

- Spontaneous birth of baby
- No prophylactic uterotonic
- Umbilical cord left unclamped
- Signs of placental separation
- Placenta delivered by maternal effort

Active management

- Birth of baby's anterior shoulder
- Administration of IM uterotonic, with consent
- Uterine contraction
- Controlled cord traction whilst guarding uterus

---

5 international units (IU) oxytocin and 0.5 mg ergometrine maleate, both belonging to the group of medicines known as oxytocics which cause the uterus to contract. The route of choice is intramuscular, and the site is often the accessible lateral aspect of the leg (Baston et al 2009). The Syntocinon component of Syntometrine works within 2 to 3 minutes and lasts only 5 to 15 minutes, whereas the ergometrine takes 6 to 7 minutes to work but has a sustained action lasting up to 2 hours (Johnson & Taylor 2006). Ergometrine can have the undesirable side-effects of nausea, vomiting, headache and raised blood pressure (Jordan 2002). If the use of ergometrine is contraindicated – for example, if the woman has hypertension – then oxytocin should be administered.

When intravenous oxytocin is required, a dose of 5 IU should be administered slowly by an experienced practitioner.

The NICE intrapartum care guidelines recommend the use of 10 international units (IU) of Syntocinon by intramuscular injection, although it is not licensed to be given by this route (Alliance Pharmaceuticals 2007). A systematic review examining the prophylactic use of oxytocin during the third stage of labour (Cotter et al 2001) concluded that oxytocin is beneficial in the prevention of PPH. However, there was insufficient evidence regarding the side-effects of its use and to what extent they compromise its use. There was little evidence to support the use of ergometrine alone versus Syntocinon alone or a combined product for preventing PPH of more than 1000 ml and the authors recommend further research to evaluate their use. A subsequent review (McDonald et al 2007) found a small reduction in PPH of 500 ml when a combined ergometrine–Syntocinon product was used, but again no difference between groups for blood loss of more than 1000 ml. The authors concluded that the undesirable effects of nausea, vomiting and raised diastolic blood pressure need to be weighed againt the reduction in blood loss.

Oral misoprostol has also been used as a means of actively managing the third stage of labour. A randomized controlled trial (Oboro & Tabowei 2003), comparing oral misoprostol with intramuscular oxytocin after birth, found no significant differences between the groups regarding postpartum haemorrhage, length of third stage or the incidence of manual removal of the placenta. However, more women experienced shivering in the misoprostol group and another study (Lumbiganon et al 2002) found that misoprostol was associated with post-delivery diarrhoea.

Activity

How many millilitres are there in a litre?
    How many micrograms are there in a milligram?
    Make sure you know in what circumstances intravenous oxytocin is given.
    Find out why misoprostol is useful in tropical conditions.

Controlled cord traction (CCT)

If an oxytocic has been administered, then the placenta and membranes are usually delivered by CCT. This technique, when applied in the UK, generally involves the midwife awaiting signs of separation (of the placenta from the uterine wall). These include: contraction of the uterus which will change from feeling broad to becoming firm and more rounded, lengthening of the cord at the introitus and a small trickle of blood observed from the vagina. A sterile towel is placed on the woman's abdomen, and the midwife places her still hand on the towel to await a contraction.

If right-handed, the midwife will 'guard' the uterus with her left hand by keeping her fingers together, opening her thumb and positioning her hand on the woman's abdomen just above the symphysis pubis. The purpose of this action is to prevent the uterus from following the placenta and prolapsing or inverting. The midwife continues to 'guard' the uterus while she undertakes CCT. Firm backward counter-pressure is applied, and this position should be maintained throughout CCT (the hand only being removed after traction has stopped).

With the right hand, the midwife takes the clamped cord and wraps it around her index and middle fingers. Firm, but slow and steady, traction is used to guide the placenta into the vagina. This traction is down towards the bed or floor, depending on the woman's position. If, as traction is applied, the midwife feels that the cord is breaking, then traction should cease and the maternal effort method should be employed.

Actively delivering the placenta and membranes

When the bulk of the placenta appears
at the vulva, the direction of traction is
changed to a horizontal then upward
movement. When the whole placenta
is visible, the midwife cups it in her
hands and slowly rotates it in a clockwise
direction, thus twisting the membranes
that follow it into a rope. This action is
undertaken with the aim of keeping the
membranes together in a form that can
conveniently be grasped with forceps
if they are reluctant to escape from
the uterus. The delivery of this rope of
membranes can be assisted by slowly
lifting the cupped placenta up then down
and up again. This action is repeated
until the membranes are completely
expelled. The placenta and membranes
are placed in the sterile receiver included
in the birth pack, to await inspection.

Physiological management

Physiological or expectant management
of third stage should only be offered
if the first and second stages were also
physiological, hence the balance of
hormonal and psychological aspects

of birth remain in equilibrium (Fry
2007). As it is often hospital policy
to undertake active management of
the third stage, many midwives will
not be confident with this aspect of
midwifery care. It is therefore rarely
offered as an option when the birth
plan is being discussed. However,
women who request a physiological
third stage should receive skilled and
competent care from the midwife
and it is important therefore that
an understanding of the principles
of physiological management are
maintained to prevent this practice from
becoming a 'dying art' (Walsh 2003).

The central principle is to observe
the process – do not intervene unless
the woman starts to bleed heavily or the
baby needs separating from the mother
for resuscitation. A small trickle of blood
from the vagina is normal as the placenta
separates. Physiological third stage can
take up to 1 hour, although the average
length of time in the Hinchingbrooke
trial for physiological management was
15 minutes (Rogers & Wood 1999).
Constant attention and observation
must be maintained. The woman should
not be left by the midwife while the
placenta is still in utero.

Maternal effort

If the woman has not had an oxytocic, and a 'hands-off' approach is being taken, she can wait until she feels the placenta in her vagina and then simply push it out. An upright sitting, kneeling or squatting position will work with gravity to assist this process. If the membranes remain in the vagina, the midwife should use the twisting method described above to ensure their complete expulsion.

If maternal effort is being used because CCT had to be abandoned (because the cord was thin, weak or was felt to be shearing from the placenta), and the woman has had an oxytocic, she should be encouraged to bear down. She may find this activity a little difficult or strange after her exertions during the second stage. She may benefit from you placing a flat hand on her abdomen and asking her to push against your hand.

Delivering the placenta after caesarean birth

A range of methods for delivering the placenta following surgical birth have been practised including manual removal, spontaneous delivery after placental drainage and cord traction. A systematic review of the research evidence (Anorlu et al 2008) concluded that cord traction results in fewer complications including less blood loss and associated reduction in haematocrit, less endometritis and shorter hospital stay.

Cutting the cord

Increasingly, parents are requesting involvement in this significant aspect of the birth of their baby. It is a request that can usually be accommodated, even if the baby is born by forceps or ventouse extraction. The obstetrician or instrumental practitioner should be made aware at the beginning of the delivery and then gently reminded as the baby is born. It is important to respect and accommodate where possible the details of the parents' aspirations for the birth. These form part of the story that will be told for many years to come.

Before the cord is cut, it must be clamped. A pair of cord clamps is included in the delivery pack, and checked and positioned within easy reach of the midwife. Once the baby is born and safely in its mother's arms, the central part of the cord is identified and the left hand placed underneath it (so that no other parts of the anatomy are inadvertently grasped) before a clamp is secured. (You will become familiar with the sound and feel of cord clamps that have been correctly secured; they make a characteristic crunch as the ratchets engage.) Then, holding the clamp in the right hand, take the cord to the left of the clamp and firmly squeeze it between index finger and thumb back towards the woman for a few centimetres. Keeping the left hand firm and letting go of the first clamp, pick up the second clamp and secure it just in front of your thumb. This process should result in a section of cord that is white because the blood has been squeezed out. This is where the cord can be cut without anyone being sprayed with blood. Although a long process to describe, it takes seconds to perform and is a practice well worth becoming adept at. The cord is cut with specially designed scissors which are short with a characteristically circular blade.

Examination of the genital tract following the birth

Following the complete expulsion of the placenta and membranes, the time is noted so that it can be documented on the partogram. It is then important to examine the woman's vagina and external genitalia for trauma. This is not a pleasant procedure for the woman and if it is known that suturing will almost certainly be required (because there is an obvious second-degree tear or episiotomy) this examination can be delayed until the woman has had analgesia. However, if she is bleeding from her vagina continuously and the uterus is contracted, it will be necessary to identify where the bleeding is coming from.

An explanation of the purpose of this examination should precede gaining verbal consent. The woman should be informed that you would like to see if she needs any stitches and that you will be looking inside her vagina and at her perineum. If she is tense then it will be difficult to undertake the examination. She may benefit from some Entonox to help her relax. If she is holding her baby at this point, then the partner can hold

the baby close so that the woman can see him/her.

A good, focused light source is required, but it need not be intrusive. Using the left-hand finger and thumb to part the labia, take a sterile cotton swab between the index and middle fingers of the right hand and gently insert into the vagina. If the swab becomes soaked with blood, replace and ensure that the uterus remains firm so that the field is clear from trickling blood. Examine the lateral and posterior vaginal walls for lacerations. Then examine the vulva and perineum. See Chapter 11 for perineal suturing technique.

Post-birth observations

Clinical observation

In order to establish that the woman has not been physically compromised as a result of the birth, observations of temperature, pulse and blood pressure should be taken within the first hour of birth. All observations should be documented on the partogram, and any deviation from the norm reported to a senior midwife.

It is important to ensure that the uterus remains contracted. With permission, a hand should be placed on the woman's abdomen to ensure that the uterus is firm and central and below the level of the umbilicus. After birth, the uterus is traditionally described as feeling like a cricket ball – that is, very firm. If the uterus feels soft, broad or spongy, a contraction should be 'rubbed up'.

This involves placing a hand on the uterine fundus and, keeping the fingers in the same position, making a rapid circular movement until the uterus is felt to respond by becoming firm again. The woman should be informed of what you are doing and why. If the uterus feels high or deviated to either side, then this may be because a full bladder is displacing it. The woman should be encouraged to pass urine if she can.

Again, with the woman's permission, her sanitary pad should be checked to observe her blood loss. The pad should be changed before it becomes soaked. Uterine tone and blood loss should be checked regularly following birth, especially in this first hour.

Examination of the placenta

The most important reason for examining the placenta is for completeness, to ascertain whether any of it might potentially remain within the uterus. The woman should be asked if she wants to see her placenta and, additionally, if she wants to see it examined.

The examination should be systematic so that you develop a way of performing it that helps you remember each aspect. Starting from the cord end, take hold of the clamp and wipe away any blood from the cut end. There are two arteries and a vein (remembered using the AVA acronym). Occasionally there is only one artery in the cord and this should be recorded and reported to the paediatrician. A renal ultrasound may be requested to exclude renal agenesis.

Looking carefully at the end section of the cord, it is possible to see two small circles (the transverse section of the umbilical arteries). The vein is larger but sometimes more difficult to distinguish as its walls are more floppy and likely to have flattened. Moving along the cord, the midwife notes its place of insertion into the placenta, which is usually central or slightly to one side. This fetal side of the placenta is pale and shiny.

Then, turning the placenta over, the maternal side is explored. The red-raw surface of it should be examined by running a flat (gloved!) hand across it. Sometimes it feels gritty due to lime salt deposition, however, this is insignificant (Johnson & Taylor 2006). This surface comprises 15–20 cotyledons, which should all fit neatly in apposition with each other. If there is a gap, it is possible that a cotyledon has been retained in the uterus – this should be recorded on the partogram and reported to a senior midwife.

On examination of the membranes, the hole through which the baby was born should be identifiable, and it will be possible to separate the amnion (fetal side) from the chorion (maternal side). If the membranes are ragged, then it may be possible that a fragment has been retained – again, this should be noted and reported.

Estimating blood loss

Assessing blood loss following birth is acknowledged to be subjective and

Activity

Define a velamentous insertion of the cord.

Define a battledore insertion.

Describe what action would be taken if the placenta appeared incomplete on examination.

Find out how much the placenta normally weighs. Why might it be smaller or larger?

Activity

List the precautions taken by the midwife to avoid contact with body fluids when caring for a woman in labour.

Write down the reasons why episiotomy scissors should not be used for cutting the umbilical cord.

fraught with difficulties. It soaks into the bed sheets and is mixed with liquor. Razvi et al (1996) compared visual estimation of blood loss with laboratory estimation and concluded that visual estimation is inaccurate, particularly at extremes of blood loss and that it is not an accurate means of detecting postpartum haemorrhage. Prasertcharoensuk et al (2000) support the stance that visual estimation results in underestimation of blood loss. Hence, all attempts should be made to enhance this estimation, by gathering clots and blood from the birth into a measuring jug. It can only ever be an estimation, which should be recorded on the partogram.

Wickham (1999) observes that, in her experience, women who have a physiological third stage may lose more blood at birth (that is noted and recorded) but that women who have active management are more likely to have minimal blood loss immediately after the birth but then go on to lose more blood when the effect of the oxytocic has worn off.

Variations on a theme

Occasionally, a physiological third stage may have been planned but the cord was cut after the birth of the head because the cord was around the neck. The cord might also have been cut if there was meconium-stained liquor or the baby needed resuscitation. The woman might wish to continue without an oxytocic and expel the placenta with maternal effort.

Active management of third stage can involve more intervention than is common practice in the UK. For example, Jackson et al (2001) describe the management of third stage in their unit in North Carolina whereby a bolus of intravenous oxytocics is given after the placenta has been delivered by CCT. This is followed by bimanual fundal massage for 15 seconds. In a randomized controlled trial comparing this method with an IV bolus of oxytocin commenced at the birth of the fetal anterior shoulder, they found no differences between the groups for third-stage duration or PPH. The incidence of retained placenta was not increased by early administration of intravenous oxytocin.

Some women feel that they would like to have a natural third stage but are not prepared to be totally hands-off. A compromise may be agreed whereby the midwife waits until the cord stops pulsating and then gives Syntometrine. Alternatively, they can wait and see how it goes with the advantage of having drugs to hand if required.

This would seem an ideal solution for those with limited experience. However, babies who do not have their umbilical cord clamped and severed immediately after they are born can behave differently from those who continue to receive oxygenated blood from the placenta. They are slower to cry as one of the stimuli to breathe is 'the gradual cessation of the baby's oxygen supply from the placenta via the cord after birth' (Long 2003:369). For midwives who are unaccustomed to observing this normal process, this delay might appear to be evidence that the baby requires assistance, resulting in clamping and cutting the cord in order to administer oxygen. Thus, midwives must be conversant with all aspects of physiological management and be able to recognize both neonatal and maternal compromise in order to provide effective care.

Another approach is to avoid giving oxytocics, observe for signs of separation and then use CCT and maternal effort to deliver the placenta (Reynolds et al 2002:218). Reynolds asserts that midwives '…have developed styles of third-stage management that are appropriate to different clinical situations and individual women's needs and values, a hallmark of midwifery care.'

A less common approach to third stage is the practice 'lotus birth' which involves keeping the placenta attached by the cord to the baby until it separates naturally (Crowther 2006). The cord is not clamped or cut and the washed and wrapped placenta is kept in a bag alongside the baby.

Prolonged third stage

The third stage of labour is said to be prolonged after 30 minutes of the birth of the baby if active management was employed and after 60 minutes of the birth if expectant management was the chosen method (NICE 2007:33).

Tips to help expel the placenta
Breastfeeding

Putting the baby to the breast soon after birth should be encouraged for all women. When there is delay in expulsion of the placenta, the natural release of oxytocin by the woman during breastfeeding can assist the uterus to contract and the placenta to shear away from the uterine wall.

Maternal position

Upright positions work with gravity to assist expulsion of the placenta. Sitting on a bedpan on a chair, kneeling, squatting or standing are all useful alternatives.

Empty the bladder

If the urinary bladder is full, then the placenta may be prevented from being delivered. If the woman is unable to pass urine herself, then it will be necessary to use a urinary catheter.

Retained placenta

There is no consistent evidence that either method of management of the third stage predisposes to retained placenta (Brucker 2001). The woman should be kept up-to-date with the situation so that she knows what to expect. A doctor will be informed, and preparations made for manual removal of the placenta. An intravenous infusion will be started. If the woman does not have an epidural in situ, she will be advised that this is the anaesthetic of choice, otherwise she will require general anaesthesia.

The procedure is undertaken by a doctor who will locate a separated edge of the placenta with the right hand and, with the palm facing the placenta, gently peel it away from the wall of the uterus. The left hand supports the fundus abdominally and is used to rub up a contraction. When the placenta is totally separated, the right hand is removed holding the placenta. An oxytocic drug will then be given – usually by slow, continuous infusion – and the placenta examined for completeness. Prophylactic antibiotics are normally prescribed to avoid the development of puerperal sepsis (Lindsay 2004).

If a retained placenta is diagnosed at home, the woman should not be moved until an intravenous infusion has been started. She should be transferred to hospital with her baby, by paramedic ambulance (or locally agreed alternative).

Activity

Describe the potential causes of postpartum haemorrhage.

List the risks associated with retained placenta.

Define placenta accreta, and describe how it is managed.

Find out about bimanual compression of the uterus, and when it is indicated.

Disposal of the placenta

The placenta belongs to the woman. However, most are happy for it to be incinerated at the hospital. When the woman has had a home birth, the midwife must attend to careful disposal of the placenta, in accordance with local policy. This may involve the use of a special 'placenta bucket' with a sealable lid, but is more likely to be the use of double bagging in yellow human waste bags. The placenta will then be transported in the midwife's car back to the maternity unit for disposal in the same manner as for hospital births.

If the baby was stillborn (either at home or in hospital), it is often requested that the placenta should be sent to the laboratory for detailed histological investigation. It is essential that the appropriate completed histology form accompanies the placenta. Parents should always be involved and informed about possible tests and samples taken from their baby.

Documentation

This is one time when it is appropriate to complete documentation away from the woman and partner, allowing them private time to explore their new baby. The midwife should ensure that they know how to call for assistance if required and the woman should not be left unattended holding the baby if she is ill, sedated or very tired. The midwife must complete the partogram indicating how third stage was managed and at what time it was completed. Examination of the placenta, estimation of blood loss, perineal trauma and post-birth observations should all be documented.

Reflection on trigger

Look back on the trigger scenario.

The midwife wiped Liz's face with a cool flannel. 'Did you want to push with that contraction?' she asked. Liz kept her eyes closed and nodded. The gas and air was just wearing off. 'We'd better get ready then,' the midwife said. She turned to the student, 'Just check this Syntometrine for me.' Turning to the woman, she said, 'Are you happy to have the injection in your leg for the afterbirth?' But Liz was using the gas and air. Another contraction had started.

Now that you are familiar with the principles of third stage care you should have insight into how the scenario relates to the evidence. The jigsaw model will now be used to explore the trigger scenario in more depth.

Effective communication

The midwife and woman need to communicate effectively so that information can change hands to inform discussions about the most appropriate management of care. With regard to the third stage, such discussion should ideally have taken place during pregnancy, to enable Liz and her partner to consider the options available. Questions that arise from the scenario might include: What does Liz already know about the third stage of labour? How might the midwife have re-phrased the question about Syntometrine so as not to direct Liz's response?

Woman-centred care

For women to be central to the decisions about their care they need to have access to unbiased evidence in a format they can understand. They need to have time to weigh up what might be the best approach for them according to their individual circumstances. What might be a simple decision for one woman may be complicated by previous experience, culture, health and social circumstances for another. Questions that arise from the scenario might include: Had Liz had Syntometrine during a previous birth? If so, how had she made that decision and what had been the effects? How else can the midwife find out what the woman felt about having an oxytocic drug to reduce the length of the third stage of labour?

Using best evidence

To make an informed decision about whether or not to use oxytocic drugs for the third stage the woman needs information about the relative advantages and disadvantages of each method. Information should reflect what is known about a particular course of action as well as the gaps in our understanding and midwives need to develop their skills in informing women of their choices (Kanikosamy 2007). Whilst a particular course of action may have some benefits it may also have undesirable side-effects. Questions that arise from the scenario might include: In what circumstances is Syntometrine contraindicated? Has Liz been informed of the side-effects of Syntometrine? What are the optimum storage conditions for Syntometrine? What are the consequences of storing Syntometrine outside of these conditions?

Professional and legal issues

Establishing whether an individual has the capacity to give consent is a complex issue, supported by a detailed legal framework. Midwives must ensure that they practise within the law and in accordance with professional standards and locally agreed guidelines. Questions that arise from the scenario might include: Is the woman able to give consent for a drug when she is using Entonox? How can the midwife demonstrate that she was working in the woman's best interests if she gives Syntometrine in these circumstances? What are the possible consequences of giving a drug without consent? In what circumstances can a student midwife administer drugs?

Team working

Whether the midwife is supporting a woman to give birth at home or in the hospital environment, she is dependent on a range of people for support and should work to develop and maintain effective working relationships with all members of the multi-disciplinary team. Questions that arise from the scenario might include: Whom should the midwife inform if Liz does not birth her placenta within 1 hour following a physiological approach to third stage? Which professionals might subsequently become involved in Liz's care? If Liz was having a home birth, who else might contribute to Liz's care? If Liz needed to go to theatre for manual removal of her placenta, who else would be involved in her care?

Clinical dexterity

Caring for women during the third stage of labour requires the midwife to have developed a high degree of clinical dexterity. In order to perform these skills she needs a sound knowledge of the theory behind what she is doing. The midwife needs to know when to abandon one course of action in favour of another and how to involve the woman throughout the process. Questions that arise from the scenario might include: How can the midwife encourage the woman to birth her own placenta? In what circumstances should controlled cord traction be used to deliver the placenta? When should maternal effort be used instead of CCT during an actively managed third stage? Where is the most appropriate site for administering

Syntometrine in a woman who is giving birth in the left lateral position?

Models of care

The care a woman receives may be influenced by the model of care that she has chosen or that has been made available to her. For example, midwives caring for women in consultant-led units may be expected to follow guidelines that promote the active management of the third stage, whereas women cared for in a midwife-led unit or by an independent midwife may take a more liberal approach. Ideally, guidelines should be written with the involvement of midwives and women, that enable midwives to exercise clinical judgment within an evidence-based framework, and women to make choices that meet their aspirations for birth. Questions that arise from the scenario might include: Where was Liz giving birth? How might place of birth influence care during the third stage of labour? What systems are in place to ensure that midwifery care guidelines facilitate informed choice for women and support the provision of safe care in all settings?

Safe environment

Midwives should ensure that they keep up-to-date with changes in clinical practice and refresh their knowledge in aspects of care they do not come across on a regular basis. Therefore, to offer safe care for women with regard to a physiological third stage, midwives who work within an environment where active management is the norm need to ensure that they are able to undertake a physiological third stage for women who request it. Questions that arise from the scenario might include: What opportunities are there where you work to discuss issues such as physiological third stage with experienced midwives? Are the outcomes and management methods for third stage audited on a regular basis? When oxytocic drugs are used, how can the midwife ensure that the correct drug and dose is prepared for administration? What safety measures should the midwife follow to ensure that s/he gives the right drug to the right person? How can the midwife minimize the risk of needle stick injury whilst administering intramuscular injections to women in labour? How are placentas disposed of where you work?

Promotes health

The midwife must be vigilant during third stage of labour, whichever method is being used. She can promote the sense of wellbeing in the woman by facilitating the method of her choice with confidence and competence. By practising safely the midwife can minimize the risk of excessive blood loss and respond quickly if the woman's condition deviates from normal. Questions that arise from the scenario might include: What are the training opportunities where you work for the management of postpartum haemorrhage due to retained placenta? What are the side-effects of giving Syntometrine? In what circumstances would it be advantageous for the woman to agree to an actively managed third stage of labour?

Further scenarios

The following scenarios enable you to consider how specific situations influence the care the midwife provides. Use the jigsaw model to explore the issues raised in the scenario.

Scenario 1

Julie is 20 weeks pregnant and would like to birth her baby at home. With her second baby, the placenta was retained and it was documented in her notes that it had been 'placenta accreta'. Her community midwife has arranged for Julie to discuss her aspirations for home birth with the consultant obstetrician.

Practice point

There is no legal requirement that women should come into hospital to birth their babies. It is important therefore that the midwife establishes and maintains a trusting relationship with Julie so that they can work together to identify the most suitable course of action. Julie should not be coerced in any way, but should be presented with information in such a way that enables her to make an appropriate choice. All options should be considered whereby a safe plan of care can be adopted.

Further questions specific to Scenario 1 include:

1. What is placenta accreta?
2. What are the chances of this happening again in a subsequent pregnancy?
3. How is placenta accreta managed?
4. What issues would the consultant be likely to raise when s/he meets Julie?

5. How can the community midwife help Julie achieve a safe and satisfactory experience of birth?
6. What particular preparations should be made for the birth of Julie's second baby?

Scenario 2

Emma has just given birth to her third baby and has requested a physiological third stage of labour. Both her previous births involved interventions and she would really like to see if her body can birth her baby and placenta unaided. However, 40 minutes after the birth of the baby there is no sign of the placenta.

Practice point

Whilst delivering placentas may be an everyday event for midwives working on the labour ward, for most women it will be something they do two or three times in their lifetime. For many women, third stage is an unimportant aspect of the birthing process and not one that they have given much thought to. However, some women are keen to experience a birth without drugs or intervention and this includes the birth of the placenta.

Further questions specific to Scenario 2 include:

1. Where did the woman give birth?
2. What action can the midwife suggest to help facilitate a physiological third stage?
3. What is the average length of a physiological third stage?

4. What clinical maternal observations should the midwife be making following the birth of the baby?

5. What are the risks associated with a prolonged third stage of labour?

6. Whom can the midwife call to her aid if the placenta remains undelivered?

Conclusion

Active management is the most prevalent form of third-stage care. It is most effective for reducing the incidence of PPH, and reduces the length of third stage. It is, however, associated with nausea, vomiting and raised blood pressure, and all of these aspects should be explored with the woman to enable her to make a choice that is right for her. Whichever method she chooses, the midwife must be able to provide safe and supportive care based on his/her knowledge of normal physiology.

Resources

Association of Radical Midwives. Third stage of labour and postpartum haemorrhage: http://www.radmid. demon.co.uk/pph.htm.

Home birth reference site: third stage of labour: http://www.homebirth.org. uk/thirdstage.htm.

Joint statement of management of the third stage of labour to prevent postpartum haemorrhage. International Confederation of Midwives (ICM)/International Federation of Gynaecologists and Obstetricians (FIGO): http://www.figo.org/docs/ PPH%20Joint%20Statement.pdf.

Women's Health Specialist library: third stage of labour: http://www.library. nhs.uk/womenshealth/ViewResource. aspx?resID=82612.

References

Alliance Pharmaceuticals Electronic medicines compendium: Syntocinon, 2007. Online. Available http://emc. medicines.org.uk/emc/assets/c/html/ DisplayDoc.asp?DocumentID=1642 4#CATEGORY July 20, 2008.

Anderson T: Active versus expectant management of the third stage of labour, *The Practising Midwife* 2(2):10–11, 1999.

Anorlu RI, Maholwana B, Hofmeyr GJ: Methods of delivering the placenta at caesarean section DOI: 10.1002/14651858.CD004737.pub2, *Cochrane Database of Systematic Reviews* 3(CD004737), 2008.

Baston H, Hall J, Henley-Einion A: *Midwifery essentials: basics*, Edinburgh, 2009, Elsevier.

Brucker M: Management of the third stage of labor: an evidence-based approach, *Journal of Midwifery & Women's Health* 46(6):381–392, 2001.

Combs C, Laros RJ: Prolonged third stage of labor: morbidity and risk factors, *Obstetrics and Gynecology* 77:863–867, 1991.

Cotter A, Ness A, Tolosa J: Prophylactic oxytocin for the third stage of labour DOI: 10.1002/14651858.CD001808, *Cochrane Database of Systematic Reviews* 4(CD001808):16, 2001.

Crowther S: Lotus birth: leaving the cord alone, *The Practising Midwife* 9(6):12–14, 2006.

Dombrowski M, Bottoms S, Saleh A, et al: Third stage of labour: analysis of duration and clinical practice, *American Journal of Obstetrics & Gynecology* 172:1279–1284, 1995.

Fry J: Physiological third stage of labour: support it or lose it, *British Journal of Midwifery* 15(11):693–695, 2007.

Harding J, Elbourne D, Prendiville W: Views of mothers and midwives participating in the Bristol randomized controlled trial of active management of the third stage of labour, *Birth* 16(1):1–6, 1989.

Jackson K, Allbert J, Schemmer G, et al: A randomized controlled trial comparing oxytocin administration before and after placental delivery in the prevention of postpartum hemorrhage, *American Journal of Obstetrics & Gynecology* 185(4):873–877, 2001.

Johnson R, Taylor W: *Skills for midwifery practice*, ed 2, Edinburgh, 2006, Elsevier.

Jordan S: *Pharmacology for midwives – the evidence base for safe practice*, Basingstoke, 2002, Palgrave.

Kanikosamy F: Third stage: the why of physiological practice, *Midwives* 10(9):422–425, 2007.

Kinmond S, Aitchison T, Holland B, et al: Umbilical cord clamping and preterm infants: a randomised trial, *British Medical Journal* 306(6871): 172–175, 1993.

Lindsay P: Complications of the third stage of labour. In Henderson C, Macdonald S, editors: *Mayes' Midwifery. A text book for midwives*, ed 13, Edinburgh, 2004, Baillière Tindall.

Long L: Defining third stage of labour care and discussing optimal practice, *MIDIRS Midwifery Digest* 13(3): 366–370, 2003.

Lumbiganon P, Villar J, et al: Side effects of oral misoprostol during the first 24 hours after administration in the third stage of labour, *British Journal of Obstetrics and Gynaecology* 109(11):1222–1226, 2002.

McDonald SJ, Abbott JM, Higgins SP: Prophylactic ergometrine-oxytocin versus oxytocin for the third stage of labour DOI: 10.1002/14651858. CD000201.pub2, *Cochrane Database of Systematic Reviews* 2(CD000201), 2007.

McDonald SJ, Middleton P: Effect of timing of umbilical cord clamping of term infants on maternal and neonatal outcomes DOI: 10.1002/14651858. CD004074.pub2, *Cochrane Database of Systematic Reviews* 2 (CD004074):16, 2008.

National Institute for Health and Clinical Excellence (NICE): *Intrapartum care. Care of healthy women and their* babies during childbirth. NICE clinical guideline 55, London, 2007, NICE.

Oboro V, Tabowei T: A randomised controlled trial of misoprostol versus oxytocin in the active management of the third stage of labour, Journal of Obstetrics & Gynaecology 23(1):13–16, 2003.

Prasertcharoensuk W, Swadpanich U, Lumbiganon P: Accuracy of the blood loss estimation in the third stage of labour, International Journal of Gynaecology & Obstetrics 71:69–70, 2000.

Prendiville W, Harding J, Elbourne D, et al: The Bristol third stage trial: active versus physiological management of third stage of labour, British Medical Journal 297:1295–1300, 1988.

Prendiville WJP, Elbourne D, McDonald SJ: Active versus expectant management in the third stage of labour DOI: 10.1002/14651858.CD000007, Cochrane Database of Systematic Reviews 1(CD000007), 2000.

Razvi K, Chua S, Arulkumaran S, et al: A comparison between visual estimation and laboratory determination of blood loss during the third stage of labour, Australian and New Zealand Journal of Obstetrics and Gynaecology 36(2): 152–154, 1996.

Reynolds D, Singer J, Hodgman D: Letter to the Editor, Journal of Midwifery & Women's Health 47(3): 218, 2002.

Rogers J, Wood J, McCandlish R, et al: Active versus expectant management of third stage of labour: the Hinchingbrooke randomised controlled trial, The Lancet 351(9104): 693–699, 1998.

Rogers J, Wood J: The Hinchingbrooke third stage trial. What are the implications for practice?, The Practising Midwife 2(2):35–37, 1999.

Walsh D: Haemorrhage and the third stage of labour, British Journal of Midwifery 11(2):72, 2003.

Wickham S: Further thoughts on the third stage, The Practising Midwife 2(10):14–15, 1999.

Chapter 10

Caesarean birth

Introduction

The caesarean section rate in the UK has almost doubled in recent years, from 12% in 1990 to 21% in 2000. Between 2005 and 2006, 23.5% of births were by caesarean section, and more than half of these were emergency caesareans (The Information Centre 2007). With more than one-fifth of babies being born in this way, midwives can play a key role in making the experience a positive one for women and their families. This chapter describes care around the time of the birth; postoperative and postnatal care following caesarean section is discussed in volume 4 in this series.

Terminology

An elective or planned caesarean is one that is performed during pregnancy, before the onset of labour. An emergency caesarean is one that is performed during labour. However, these definitions seem inadequate when one considers the many permutations that can occur.

For example, a woman may be admitted to the labour ward from antenatal clinic for caesarean section following ultrasonography that suggests the fetus has stopped growing and requires prompt delivery – technically an 'elective' procedure. Alternatively, a woman might be in labour but not progressing and a decision made that the only option is caesarean, although neither she nor the baby is showing signs of compromise. Her 'emergency caesarean' takes place 2 hours later.

In order to provide a more precise definition of caesarean birth, a group of anaesthetists practising in the UK (Lucas et al 2000), developed and evaluated a classification system based on the use of four grades (Table 10.1). This classification was used in the Sentinel Audit (Thomas & Paranjothy 2001:49) and The House of Commons Health Committee (2003) recommended its continued use.

Risk factors and indications for caesarean birth

In response to concerns about the rising caesarean birth rate in the United Kingdom, the National Sentinel Caesarean Birth Audit was undertaken by the Royal College of Obstetricians and Gynaecologists (Thomas & Paranjothy 2001). In addition to the collection of clinical data, women and obstetricians were surveyed about their views of childbirth, including their priorities for maternity care. One of the aims of the audit was to explore the determinants of caesarean birth. It concluded that the main primary indications for caesarean as reported by clinicians were: presumed fetal compromise (22%), failure to progress in labour (20%) and previous caesarean (14%). The caesarean birth rate was 88% for breech presentations and 59% for twin pregnancies.

Age

The National Sentinel Caesarean Birth Audit (Thomas & Paranjothy 2001) also found that women were more likely to have a caesarean birth with advancing maternal age: only 7% of women under 20 years old had a caesarean compared with 17% of women who were over 35

Table 10.1 Classification of urgency of caesarean birth

Grade	Definition
(1) Emergency	Immediate threat to life of woman or fetus
(2) Urgent	Maternal or fetal compromise which is not immediately life threatening
(3) Scheduled	Needing early delivery but no maternal or fetal compromise
(4) Elective	At a time to suit the woman and maternity team

(Lucas et al 2000, p. 349)

years old. Weaver et al (2001) argue that the perception that older women are more likely to experience complications during labour could give rise to 'an increased willingness' (p. 284) of both women and obstetricians to proceed to a caesarean.

Ethnicity

It has been reported (Tuck et al 1983) that black women (African and Caribbean) have a higher incidence of emergency caesarean birth compared with white women. Findings from the National Sentinel Caesarean Birth Audit concluded that the proportion of caesarean births was higher for women who were black African (31%) or black Caribbean (24%) compared with white women (21%). The indications for caesarean birth in these women were explored and were seen to relate to a higher proportion of maternal medical disease and fetal distress.

Primigravidae

Parity is also a significant factor in the incidence of caesarean birth. The results of the National Sentinel Audit showed that the primary caesarean birth rate in England was 24% for primigravid women and 10% for multiparous women. Of the women who had a previous caesarean the repeat caesarean rate was 67%.

Socio-economic status

Social class is also a predictor of caesarean birth. Using the index of multiple deprivation 2000, Barley

et al (2004) found that women living in the most deprived areas of England had significantly reduced odds (0.86) of having an elective caesarean birth when compared with more affluent women. There were no differences for emergency caesarean. In a prospective longitudinal study involving a cohort of 22 948 women, Hall et al (1989) found that women in social class I–IIIa (measured by the husband's occupation) were significantly more likely to have had a caesarean for the birth of their first baby than other women.

Maternal request

Maternal request has often been cited as a reason for the increase in the caesarean birth rate (Devendra & Arulkumaran 2003, Singer 2004, Singh et al 2004). According to the clinicians in the National Sentinel Caesarean Birth Audit, it accounted for 7% of caesarean births (Thomas & Paranjothy 2001:17). However, results from the maternal survey revealed that 5.3% of women would prefer a caesarean birth, and these comprised mainly women who had already had a baby by this method (op. cit. p. 95).

Thus, women rarely request, and obstetricians rarely agree to, caesarean for non-medical reasons (McCourt et al 2007). Of those that do, fear for their baby or themselves is an influential factor (Weaver et al 2007). A systematic review of caesarean for non-medical reasons (Lavender et al 2006) found no trials that could provide evidence regarding the risks and benefits of caesarean where there was no medical indication. The authors concluded that alternative research methods are used to explore the outcomes associated with different modes of birth. The decision to undertake surgical delivery should only follow full discussion of the risks and benefits for the individual woman.

Summary of indications for caesarean birth

Emergency caesarean section

Caesarean during labour may be indicated if labour is obstructed, does not progress, if there is evidence of fetal compromise, cord prolapse, antepartum haemorrhage or evidence of scar dehiscence. Where it is becoming likely that labour might end in surgery, the woman should be informed of the possibility that she might need to go to theatre. She can begin to prepare herself for this eventuality, thus preventing the ultimate decision coming as a total shock.

Elective caesarean section

Indications vary depending on individual circumstances, but include: breech presentation, previous caesarean, placenta praevia, multiple pregnancy (three or more), intrauterine growth restriction, symphysis pubis dysfunction and antepartum haemorrhage. Occasionally, it is considered necessary to undertake an elective caesarean if the woman has had a previous

traumatic experience or when a vaginal birth would almost certainly lead to psychological sequelae. Maternal request is not an indication for elective caesarean (NICE 2004).

Activity

Think about the rationale for offering elective caesarean section to women whose babies present by the breech.
   How could the incidence of such surgery be reduced?

Midwifery care

Involvement

When the situation does not go according to plan, it becomes particularly important that the woman's hopes and wishes for the birth are heeded. There may be no reason, for example, why she cannot have skin-to-skin contact with the baby after the birth or why the father should not be the one to tell her the sex of the baby. Even in the most rushed of situations, the woman can still be involved in decisions about her care. Although the situation may be out of her control, she should not be made to feel that she is having things done to her without her knowledge or consent.

As long ago as 1980, Stichler & Affonso wrote: 'The caesarean delivery is a birthing experience and must be viewed as such by all who assist the couple in the realization of their dreams.' (p. 468).

Preparation for theatre

The woman will need to be informed exactly why surgery is considered the most appropriate means of birthing the baby safely (RCOG 2006). Her verbal consent should be sought through discussion before she is asked to sign a consent form. If the woman is healthy it is not necessary to routinely take blood for 'group and save' (NICE 2004). If, however, the woman is unwell, then blood would be taken for cross-match and urgent full blood count (FBC).

It is essential that the urinary bladder is empty prior to surgery to avoid the risk of it being damaged during surgery (NICE 2004). A urinary catheter needs to be inserted, with every effort made to maintain privacy and dignity. If a regional anaesthetic needs to be administered and there is sufficient time, catheterization can be delayed until the anaesthetic has taken effect. Pubic hair needs shaving off, but not between the legs. If the woman is having elective surgery, she can do this shave herself. A clean gown is required if time permits. Jewellery should be removed and either given back to the woman's partner or taken for safe keeping as per hospital policy. Wedding rings can be taped so that they do not form a point of contact for diathermy equipment. An intravenous infusion (IVI) would be sited.

Many maternity units have implemented guidelines for thromboprophylaxis, following the recommendations of an RCOG working party (1995), and ask all women who

are likely to be immobile for some time to wear anti-embolic stockings. Thrombosis and thromboembolism account for 31% of all direct maternal deaths and are the major cause of death (Lewis 2007). If time allows, these stockings can be fitted prior to surgery, following appropriate leg measurement.

Activity

List the risk factors for thromboembolism. Find out what prophylactic measures are recommended for women undergoing caesarean birth where you work.

The woman should continue to be informed, and permission sought, before anything is done to her. She should understand why procedures are undertaken, and be introduced to anyone who comes into the room. Her birth partner should also be involved in all explanations and preparations.

In theatre

Anaesthesia for birth

Positive perceptions of caesarean section are associated with regional anaesthesia (Fawcett et al 1992, Reichert et al 1993). In the period 2005–2006, only 5% of elective and fewer than 10% of emergency caesareans were performed under general anaesthetic (The Information Centre 2007). Spinal anaesthesia accounts for 67%

of elective and over 30% of emergency surgery, with a small but rising trend in combined epidural and spinal techniques (The Information Centre 2007).

Surgical techniques: incision and closure

The **Classical** incision is rarely used, and involves a longitudinal abdominal incision. This method is used if there is an anterior placenta praevia or if the gestation is less than 32 weeks, before the lower segment has developed.

The **Pfannenstiel** (bikini) incision is a curved incision made 2 cm above the symphysis pubis transversely in the natural crease just at the top of the pubic hairline. The incision in the uterus is made in the lower segment which is less vascular than the body of the uterus, leading to less blood loss and risk of rupture in subsequent pregnancy.

The **Joel-Cohen** technique is a straight cut 3 cm above the symphysis and subsequent layers opened bluntly or with scissors rather than a knife. The Joel-Cohen method is associated with improved short-term outcomes

(Hofmeyr et al 2008) but more research is needed into the long-term implications of the various methods used.

A systematic review (Dodd et al 2008) of the techniques for incision and closure of the uterus at caesarean section found that blunt dissection at the point of uterine incision is associated with a reduced mean blood loss compared with sharp dissection. It also reported that single layer closure was associated with less blood loss, less postoperative pain and a reduced duration of procedure, but that further research was needed in this area to compare the range of techniques employed worldwide. Non-closure of the peritoneum results in a shorter procedure with no detrimental impact on maternal morbidity or postoperative pain.

There is no conclusive evidence regarding the best way to close the maternal skin after caesarean birth: staples, subcuticular and over-skin sutures all produce similar outcomes (Alderdice et al 2003).

Antibiotic cover

To reduce the incidence of postoperative infection, prophylactic antibiotics are routinely given to women who have a caesarean birth (Small & Hofmeyr 2002). Care should be taken to ensure that the woman does not have a known allergy to them. A systematic review of the drug regimes in use (Hopkins & Small 1999) concluded that ampicillin and cephalosporins have a similar effect in reducing postpartum maternal morbidity.

The birth

If the woman has regional anaesthesia, her birth partner can be with her and they will both usually be screened from the surgeon's activities by a sterile drape. However, this may not always be the case. Robinson (2003) applauds the work of one surgeon who enables each woman to truly experience the birth by lifting her baby from the uterus. Smith et al (2008) describe how they facilitate parents watching the birth and enjoying skin-to-skin contact following a slow birth from the abdominal incision.

The woman should be reassured that the effectiveness of her anaesthesia will be checked before the surgery begins. However, she will need to know that she will feel pulling and tugging, and explanations about sounds she will hear – for example, suction of liquor – should be given. It may be possible to play her favourite music in theatre, depending on the circumstances.

When the baby is born, the woman should see it immediately and be given a running commentary if it requires paediatric attention. Once the wellbeing of the baby is assured, it should be brought back to the parents while the operation continues. Skin-to-skin contact and breastfeeding can be supported at this time if the woman wishes.

If the woman has had a general anaesthetic, the baby is often taken out to the birth partner, who should be informed of the woman's condition and that it will be at least 20 minutes before she is out of theatre.

Reflection on trigger

Look back on the trigger scenario.

Susan was being prepared for an emergency caesarean birth. She began to shake, and found it difficult to sign the consent form. She looked at her husband and said, 'I don't have to be awake do I? I don't think I'm brave enough.' The midwife took the form and turning away she said, 'Don't worry, you won't see anything.'

Now that you are familiar with the principles of surgical birth you should have insight into how the scenario relates to the evidence. The jigsaw model will now be used to explore the trigger scenario in more depth.

Effective communication

Communication between the woman and midwife is essential throughout pregnancy and labour, and particularly when events do not go according to plan. It is clear that Susan is in need of information and compassion as she is prepared to undergo major abdominal surgery. Questions that arise from the scenario might include: Did Susan attend preparation for childbirth classes and if so, was caesarean birth discussed? Did the midwife explain the procedure to Susan? How was Susan's husband involved in the preparation process? Why did the midwife turn away as she was talking and how will she be able to assess the impact of her comment?

Woman-centred care

Although caesarean birth is a surgical procedure there is often scope to ensure that it remains a fulfilling and personal experience for the new parents. Although vaginal birth may not be an option, that does not mean that every other hope or aspiration needs to be abandoned. Questions that arise from the scenario might include: How was the decision made that a caesarean birth was the most appropriate way for Susan's baby to be born? What steps has the midwife taken to understand if there is anything in particular that is concerning Susan? How can the midwife ensure that the birth remains a special and family focused event? What steps can you take to protect a woman's privacy and dignity in theatre?

Using best evidence

There are many practices that are ritualistically performed with no other justification than, 'We have always done it this way.' Students have an opportunity to really question the way that care is given, looking at practice through fresh eyes. Questions that arise from the scenario might include: Is there any evidence that wearing a clean nightdress might be a source of infection to a woman undergoing surgery? What evidence is there to support the use of face masks and surgical hats in theatre? Is there any evidence that women are likely to contaminate the sterile field if they do not have a screen separating them and the surgeon? How many women would prefer to see their baby born rather than have their view obscured by a screen?

Professional and legal issues

As a surgical procedure, it is a legal requirement that consent is sought prior to caesarean birth. However, in certain circumstances, this may not be possible and the staff involved need to be able to justify their actions as being in the woman's best interests. Questions that arise from the scenario might include: Does Susan know what she is signing? In what circumstances is it impossible to gain informed consent prior to caesarean birth? Does the woman have the right to refuse a caesarean section? Who should inform the woman about the risks and benefits of the procedure? Who is responsible for counting the swabs and instruments at the end of the procedure?

Team working

Caring for a woman in childbirth involves a team of people, the majority of whom work behind the scenes. When a woman needs to have a caesarean birth, the number of people involved in her care increases significantly and they each need to come together and fulfill their own respective aspects of care. Questions that arise from the scenario might include: When was the decision made that Susan needed to go to theatre to have her baby, and who was informed? How many different professional groups are involved in the care of a woman who needs a caesarean birth?

What is the role of the birthing partner during a surgical birth? What education and training is provided where you work for healthcare assistants who work in theatre?

Clinical dexterity

The ability of a midwife to work quickly and effectively is essential when a woman needs to be prepared for an immediate caesarean birth. S/he needs to be able to locate and use a range of clinical equipment under stressful circumstances. It is also important that she instills confidence in the woman and her partner by exuding competence and confidence at all times. Questions that arise from the scenario might include: How many procedures might the midwife need to undertake before the woman has her baby? What are the advantages and disadvantages of having a dedicated theatre team versus midwives scrubbing to assist the surgeons? What opportunities and facilities are available where you work for midwives to develop and maintain their perioperative skills?

Models of care

The woman's experience of caesarean birth may be influenced by the model of care she had chosen. If she had hoped for a home birth, the process of making the decision to transfer to hospital and then to have a surgical birth, may not have been one she had previously focused on. Similarly, transferring from a stand-alone

midwifery unit into hospital is not a journey that is contemplated with joy. However, making the short journey down the corridor, for a woman who had planned a hospital birth, can be equally traumatic if she lacks information or sensitive care. The midwife has the opportunity to convey calm reassurance whilst such changes to plans are being implemented. Questions that arise from the scenario might include: Where did Susan plan to have her baby? What had influenced her choice? What are the options for Susan regarding any subsequent labours?

Safe environment

Safety is a key issue for women when they contemplate the birth of their baby. Women not only fear for their baby's life but may also fear for their own. Partners can find it very difficult observing an emergency situation develop and feeling powerless to intervene. Questions that arise from the scenario might include: Visualize the obstetric theatre where you work: how might the environment impact on someone who has never been in hospital before? What is the caesarean birth rate where you work? What measures are in place to increase the normal birth rate? What are the potential hazards of being in an obstetric theatre? How can midwives help women and their partners feel safe during the preparation and the process of surgical birth?

Promotes health

A caesarean section is a major abdominal operation and as such has significant implications for the health of the woman as she assumes her new role as mother. There are many ways in which the midwife can contribute to a safe recovery of the woman's physical and mental health. Questions that arise from the scenario might include: What advice can the midwife give to women to help them avoid the risk of developing deep vein thrombosis in the postoperative period? How should the woman look after her abdominal wound? What strategies can the woman employ to enable her to get sufficient rest to enjoy the early days of motherhood with her new baby?

Further scenarios

The following scenarios enable you to consider how specific situations influence the care the midwife provides. Use the jigsaw model to explore the issues raised in each scenario.

Scenario 1

Vanessa was 38 weeks pregnant with her first baby and attending her local community midwifery antenatal clinic. The midwife spent a long time palpating her uterus, going back and forth from palpating the fundus to palpating the presenting part. Eventually she placed her hands calmly on Vanessa's abdomen and said, 'I think this baby is coming bottom first'.

Practice point

Approximately 3–4% of babies present by the breech at term (Johnson & Taylor 2006). This means that the midwife will regularly come across women who need information about the implications of this presentation. Most hospital trusts have guidelines that recommend elective caesarean birth for breech, however, some women want to know the evidence behind such guidance and look to their midwife to explain and justify this stance. Women also need to know about the alternatives to surgery in order to make an informed choice.

Further questions specific to Scenario 1 include:

1. How did the midwife make her diagnosis?
2. What are the alternatives to elective caesarean for breech presentation?
3. If Vanessa chose to have an elective caesarean, when would be the optimum gestation to book the surgery?
4. What are the risks for the baby associated with elective caesarean?
5. What are the implications of the rising caesarean section rate for breech presentation?

Scenario 2

Jodie was at work typing a letter for her boss. She suddenly felt her pants become warm and damp. She looked down and saw a bright red patch developing on her trousers. She slowly stood up and then sat down again, feeling quite wobbly on her legs. She turned to her colleague and said, 'I think something's wrong with the baby.'

Practice point

Fresh painless vaginal bleeding is indicative of placental abruption, an obstetric emergency associated with fetal demise and maternal morbidity. In more than two-thirds of women, bleeding is revealed; however, in the remaining third there is no apparent blood loss but uterine pain is the presenting symptom (Holmes & Baker 2006). Jodie needs prompt medical attention and is reliant on her colleagues to recognize the seriousness of the situation.

Further questions specific to Scenario 2 include:

1. What causes placental abruption?

2. How is placental abruption diagnosed?
3. What are the risks of placental abruption to the mother/fetus?
4. How should the mother's condition be stabilized?
5. What form of anaesthesia is recommended in such a case?

Conclusion

Midwives can help women look back on their experience of caesarean birth with a sense of satisfaction and achievement. Sensitive midwifery care tailored to the needs of individual women can make a difference to the way this important event is both experienced and remembered.

Resources

Birth after previous caesarean birth (Royal College of Obstetricians 2007) Green top guideline: http://www.rcog. org.uk/resources/Public/pdf/green_ top45_birthafter.pdf.

Caesarean birth and (Vaginal Birth After Caesarean) VBAC information (National Childbirth Trust): http:// caesarean.org.uk/.

Controlled drugs in perioperative care: http://www.aagbi.org/publications/ guidelines/docs/controlleddrugs06.pdf.

External cephalic version (Royal College of Obstetricians 2006) Green top

guideline 20a: http://www.rcog.org. uk/resources/Public/pdf/green_top20a_ externalcephalica.pdf.

Good practice in the management of continuous epidural in the hospital setting (Royal College of Anaesthetists// Royal College of Nursing 2004): http:// www.aagbi.org/publications/guidelines/ docs/epidanalg04.pdf.

Intraoperative cell salvage (NICE 2005): http://www.nice.org.uk/nicemedia/pdf/ ip/IPG144guidance.pdf.

References

Alderdice F, McKenna D, Dornan J: Techniques and materials for skin closure in caesarean section, *Cochrane Database of Systematic Reviews* 2(CD003577), 2003, DOI: 10.1002/14651858.CD003577.

Barley K, Aylin P, Bottle A, et al: Social class and elective caesareans in the English NHS, *British Medical Journal* 328(7453):1399, 2004.

Devendra K, Arulkumaran S: Should doctors perform an elective caesarean section on request, *Annals of the Academy of Medicine, Singapore* 32(5):577–581, 2003.

Dodd JM, Anderson ER, Gates S: Surgical techniques for uterine incision and uterine closure at the time of caesarean section, *Cochrane Database of Systematic Reviews* 3(CD004732), 2008, DOI: 10.1002/14651858.CD004732. pub2.

Fawcett J, Pollio N, Tully A: Women's perceptions of cesarean and vaginal delivery: another look, *Research in Nursing & Health* 15:439–446, 1992.

Hall MH, Campbell DM, Fraser C, et al: Mode of delivery and future fertility, *British Journal of Obstetrics & Gynaecology* 96(11):1297–1303, 1989.

Hofmeyr GJ, Mathai M, Shah AN, et al: Techniques for caesarean section, *Cochrane Database of Systematic Reviews* 1(CD004662), 2008, DOI: 10.1002/14651858.CD004662. pub2.

Holmes D, Baker P, editors: *Midwifery by ten teachers*, London, 2006, Hodder Arnold.

Hopkins L, Small F: Antibiotic prophylaxis regimens and drugs for cesarean section, *Cochrane Database of Systematic Reviews* 2(CD001136), 1999, DOI: 10.1002/14651858.CD001136.

House of Commons Health Committee: Choice in maternity services. Ninth Report of Session 2002–03, 2003.

The Information Centre: NHS maternity statistics, England: 2005–2006. Government Statistical Service, 2007. Online. Available http://www.ic.nhs. uk/webfiles/publications/maternity0506/ NHSMaternityStatsEngland200506_ fullpublication%20V3.pdf. December 11, 2008.

Johnson R, Taylor W: *Skills for midwifery practice*, ed 2, Edinburgh, 2006, Elsevier.

Lavender T, Hofmeyr GJ, Neilson JP, et al: Caesarean section for non-medical reasons at term, *Cochrane Database of Systematic Reviews* 3(CD004660), 2006, DOI: 10.1002/14651858.CD004660. pub2.

Lewis GE: The confidential enquiry into maternal and child health (CEMACH). Saving mothers' lives: reviewing maternal deaths to make motherhood safer – 2003–2005. *The seventh report on confidential enquiries into maternal deaths in the United Kingdom,* London, 2007, CEMACH.

Lucas D, Yentis S, Kinsella S, et al: Urgency of caesarean section: a new classification, *Journal of the Royal Society of Medicine* 93(7):346–350, 2000.

McCourt C, Weaver J, Statham H, et al: Elective cesarean section and decision making: a critical review of the literature, *Birth* 34(1):65–79, 2007.

National Institute for Health and Clinical Excellence (NICE): *Caesarean section. Clinical guideline 13*, London, 2004, NICE.

Reichert J, Baron M, Fawcett J: Changes in attitude towards cesarean birth, *Journal of Obstetric, Gynecologic, and Neonatal Nursing* 22:159–167, 1993.

Robinson J: Improving the caesarean experience, *British Journal of Midwifery* 11(1):48, 2003.

Royal College of Obstetricians and Gynaecologists (RCOG): *Report of a working party on prophylaxis against thromboembolism in gynaecology and obstetrics*, London, 1995, RCOG.

Royal College of Obstetricians and Gynaecologists (RCOG): Caesarean section, consent advice, 2006. Online. Available http://www.rcog.org.uk/index.asp?PageID=1633 December 11, 2008

Singer B: Elective cesarean sections gaining acceptance, *Canadian Medical Association Journal* 170(5):775, 2004.

Singh T, Justin CW, Haloob RK: An audit on trends of vaginal delivery after one previous caesarean section, *Journal of Obstetrics & Gynaecology* 24(2):135–138, 2004.

Small F, Hofmeyr GJ: Antibiotic prophylaxis for cesarean section DOI: 10.1002/14651858.CD000933, *Cochrane Database of Systematic Reviews* 1(CD000933), 2002.

Smith J, Plaat F, Fisk NM: The natural caesarean: a woman centred technique, *British Journal of Obstetrics and Gynaecology* 115(8):1037–1042, 2008.

Stichler J, Affonso D: Cesarean birth, *American Journal of Nursing* 80: 466–468, 1980.

Thomas J, Paranjothy S: *National Sentinel Caesarean Section Audit Report*, 2001, Royal College of Obstetricians and Gynaecologists Clinical Effectiveness Support Unit, RCOG Press.

Tuck S, Cardozo L, Studd J, et al: Obstetric characteristics in different racial groups, *British Journal of Obstetrics and Gynaecology* 90(10):892–897, 1983.

Weaver J, Statham H, Richards M: Are there 'unnecessary' caesarean sections? Perceptions of women and obstetricians about caesarean sections for nonclinical indications, *Birth* 34(1):32–41, 2007.

Chapter 11

Perineal repair

Trigger scenario

Penny held her baby close and kissed her forehead, breathing in her smell and warmth. Her baby was finally here. The hard work of the last countless hours had come to an end. She looked up at her husband, who was cradling them both. They exchanged smiles and explored their daughter's tiny fingers and fine dark hair. They talked to her gently. 'I'm afraid you're going to need stitches,' the midwife said.

Activity

Find out what proportion of women in the UK experience perineal trauma following spontaneous birth.

List the maternal factors which contribute to the extent of perineal trauma.

List the obstetric factors which increase the likelihood of trauma to the perineum.

Introduction

Perineal pain is a source of significant morbidity for many women following childbirth, not only in the immediate postnatal period but also in the longer term (Grant et al 2001). The skill and techniques employed by the midwife or doctor who assesses and cares for the woman following perineal trauma can have a significant impact on her recovery.

Classification of perineal and genital trauma

The perineum and genital tract are inspected for trauma as outlined in Chapter 9.

Trauma to the genital tract can be anterior (involving the labia, urethra, clitoris or anterior vaginal wall) or posterior (involving the posterior vaginal wall, perineal muscles or anal sphincters). For definitions of perineal or genital trauma see Table 11.1.

Table 11.1 Definitions of perineal or genital trauma (NICE 2007:36)

Classification of trauma	Description
First degree	Injury to the skin only
Second degree	Injury to the skin and perineal muscle but not the anal sphincter
Third degree	Injury to the perineum involving the anal sphincter complex: 3a – less than 50% of external anal sphincter (EAS) torn 3b – more than 50% of EAS torn 3c – internal anal sphincter (IAS) torn
Fourth degree	Injury to the perineum involving the anal sphincter complex (EAS and IAS) and anal epithelium

Precise classification is particularly useful for communication between attending practitioners and for audit of incidence of trauma and recovery success.

Activity

Check that you know which muscles can be damaged following a second-degree tear.

Revise which muscles are cut during a mediolateral episiotomy.

Find out who can suture the perineum.

Although student midwives receive initiation into perineal suturing during their pre-registration programme (NMC 2009), not until their competence has been verified are they able to undertake this role without supervision. Achieving competence requires careful observation of skilled practitioners and close supervised practice. There are many visual aids available to complement this process, including videos and lifelike models. Competence, once gained, requires maintenance, and midwives have a duty to keep up-to-date with new techniques and research evidence (NMC 2004).

In ideal circumstances, the practitioner who assisted at the birth should be the person to undertake the suturing, as this enhances continuity of carer (Dahlen & Homer 2008). In most maternity units there is a programme of training supporting midwives in the development of their suturing skills. However, as not all midwives work in the labour suite setting it is not appropriate that midwives who would not use this technique regularly should be expected to gain competence.

House officers working on the labour suite will already be proficient at a wide range of suturing. However, when they are allocated to the labour suite they will need to learn the specific skills and issues related to caring for women during such an intimate procedure. Midwives and doctors have much to learn from each other, and this aspect of care provides many opportunities for inter-professional learning (Dahlen & Homer 2008).

If a midwife feels that a repair of a perineal wound is beyond her expertise, she should refer to a senior obstetrician rather than to a house officer. All complicated tears (third or fourth degree) or extended episiotomies should be referred, with an honest explanation given to the woman.

Inspection of the perineum

It is usual practice to inspect the perineum for damage following delivery of the placenta and membranes. However, if an episiotomy has been performed or a large tear is evident, it would be unkind and uneccesary to spend time exploring the wound without analgesia, as suturing is inevitable. Further inspection can be made when the person undertaking the repair is ready to start the procedure. If, however, it is unclear if suturing is required, a quick but thorough inspection is indicated.

It is important to examine the vaginal wall even if the perineum appears intact.

The woman should be informed of what to expect and verbal consent gained. The midwife should use two cotton wool balls in her non-dominant hand to stem any blood flow from the cervix. Then using two cotton wool balls in her dominant hand she identifies the apex of any trauma, by inserting her two fingers high into the vagina and then working her way down to the introitus. Just after birth the vaginal wall is lax and it is possible to explore the lateral and posterior walls systematically, using the cotton wool to remove any blood that may be obscuring visability. The labia and clitoris also need to be inspected for tears and grazes. If there are bilateral grazes, it may be necessary to suture at least one side to avoid the two grazes healing together. The woman should be informed of your findings and the implications discussed with her.

To suture or not?

If examination of the perineum after the birth revealed that suturing was required, this observation should be discussed with the woman. It may be felt that a small first- or second-degree tear may not require suturing if it is not bleeding and the edges of the wounds fall closely together. However, the woman's choice and individual preference should be carefully considered. This can be a difficult time to obtain 'informed consent'. There is limited evidence about whether or not to suture perineal wounds, and women need to know this. It would be relatively easy for a midwife who preferred not to suture to convince a woman that she did not need stitches. The woman is unlikely to insist on this procedure and will probably take the midwife's advice. One Scottish trial, comparing suturing versus non-suturing of first- and second-degree tears in primigravidae (Fleming et al 2003), found no difference between the groups regarding perineal pain but found that women who were sutured had better wound approximation 6 weeks after the birth.

An alternative is to suture the muscle layer and leave the skin layer to heal naturally. This technique was explored in a large randomized controlled trial in the UK (Gordon et al 1998) and more recently in Nigeria (Oboro et al 2003). Although both trials found significantly more wound gaping up to 10 days after the birth when the skin was unsutured, they also concurred that there was significantly less dyspareunia (pain during intercourse) three months postnatally in this group.

If the wound is bleeding and/or the muscle edges do not appose then suturing is the most appropriate course of action. This should be started as soon after birth as is practical, while not interfering too much with the parents' adoration of their new baby.

Procedure for perineal repair

This is a sterile procedure and as such involves opening packs and draping the woman's legs and abdomen in sterile sheets. (Full details are provided in Box 11.1.) It is not essential for the person undertaking this procedure to require the woman to be in a lithotomy position, although it does enable the perineum to be clearly visualized. The NICE intrapartum care guidelines (NICE 2007) suggest that women should *usually* be in the lithotomy position for suturing, but this position should not be used for longer than is necessary. It is possible to suture without resorting to the lithotomy, as happens when a woman needs stitches following a home birth. The woman can position her bottom at the edge of the bed and her legs can be supported on two stools; the midwife sitting between them.

If lithotomy is the most appropriate position, then great care should be taken not to abduct the legs more than is necessary. This position makes a woman feel very exposed, and every effort should be made to ensure that her dignity is respected. Two attendants should cradle the woman's heels and bend her legs simultaneously and secure them on the inside of the lithotomy poles, if possible. To avoid calling another person into the room at this exposing time, the woman's birth partner, if fit and well, can help with this. Helping the woman into this position should only be done when the procedure is about to start, to avoid unnecessary exposure.

Anaesthesia for perineal repair

Before suturing can begin, effective perineal anaesthesia must be achieved.

Box 11.1 Procedure for perineal repair

• **Explain what the procedure will involve and obtain verbal consent**
Rationale To involve the woman in her care. To seek permission to undertake procedure

• **Ensure bedding is clean and dry**
Rationale To ensure maternal comfort and reduce the risk of skin abrasion

• **Ensure emergency drugs are in the room and check their expiry date**
Rationale To facilitate rapid response in the event of accidental administration of intraveous lignocaine

• **Identify a stable surface near the woman, on which sterile pack can be opened**
Rationale To create a sterile field that can be reached easily while suturing

• Identify and test a light source
Rationale To enhance visualization of the perineum

• Wash hands carefully
Rationale To minimize the risk of cross infection

• **Open sterile packs (which include the equipment listed in box 11.2) onto stable surface**
Rationale To ensure all necessary equipment is available for use

• **Pour warm water into a large bowl**
Rationale To prepare to swab the perineum

• **Pour obstetric cream into gallipot**
Rationale To prepare for lubrication of tampon

• Scrub hands
Rationale To prepare for sterile procedure

• **Don sterile gloves, attach needle to syringe, draw up and check (with assistant) 1% lignocaine**
Rationale To prepare for administration of local anaesthetic, before exposing the woman's perineum

• **Count swabs, check and organize equipment. attach needle to needle holder**
Rationale To confirm the number of swabs in use and that all necessary instruments are present, correct and ready for use

• **Assistant(s) helps woman into a position with her legs apart, covering them with a modesty sheet**
Rationale To prepare for clear visualization of the perineum, while maintaining the woman's dignity

• **Cover the woman's legs with sterile drapes (ask assistant to remove modesty sheet), place waterproof paper under her bottom and sterile drape across her abdomen**
Rationale To create a sterile field and reduce the risk of contamination

• **Swab perineum with cotton wool soaked in warm water (from anterior to posterior) using a new swab for each labia majora, then labia minor and finally the introitus**
Rationale To enable clear visualization of the perineal trauma and reduce the risk of wound contamination

continued

Box 11.1 Continued

• Infiltrate the perineum (see Box 11.3)
Rationale To ensure adequate anaesthesia, enabling the woman to relax and not feel any discomfort

• Dip the tampon in obstetric cream and insert gently into vault of vagina
Rationale To prevent uterine blood loss from obscuring the perineal wound

• Secure the tape of the tampon to the edge of the drape across the abdomen
Rationale To ensure that the tampon remains visible and is therefore removed following the procedure

• Using forceps, gently approximate the edges of the wound, including hymenal remnants, perineal skin, etc.
Rationale To visualize how the repair will look when finished. To assess that the repair is within the capabilities of the practitioner

• Identify the apex of the wound and insert an anchoring stitch approximately 0.5–1.0 cm above this point
Rationale To ensure that all of the wound has been visualized and that approximation of the vaginal mucosa is accurate

• Using a loose, continuous, non-locking stitch, work down the vaginal mucosa to the hymen, continue with the deep then superficial perineal muscle, and finish with subcuticular sutures to the skin if required
Rationale This technique is associated with less short-term pain than locking or interrupted sutures

• Remove vaginal tampon and check that haemostasis has been achieved

and that all wound edges are accurately apposed
Rationale To ensure that wound is not bleeding and correct alignment has been achieved

• Inform the woman that a finger will be inserted into her rectum and digitally check for sutures
Rationale To ensure that sutures have not inadvertently penetrated the rectum

• Offer and administer non-steroidal anti-inflammatory suppository, if not contraindicated
Rationale To provide effective analgesia and reduce associated swelling

• Apply sanitary pad to perineum, remove all drapes and, with assistance, return the woman's legs to the closed position and cover them with a sheet
Rationale To help the woman regain a comfortable position, maintaining her dignity

• Count all swabs and needles, disposing needles in sharps bin
Rationale To ensure no materials are left inside the woman and to avoid potential needle stick injury

• Dispose of equipment in line with COSHH requirements
Rationale To reduce the risk of infection, contamination and needle stick injury

• Inform the woman about the nature and extent of her perineal wound, offering advice regarding hygiene and analgesia

continued

Box 11.1 Continued

Rationale To involve the woman in her care and optimize the healing process

- **Complete detailed documentation**

Rationale To record the extent and method of repair. To record the retrieval of all swabs. To record the administration of drugs and advice given

---

Box 11.2 Equipment for perineal suturing

- Good light source
- Stable table or trolley
- Sterile suture pack (contents: 2 bowls for water and lubricant, cotton wool, sanitary pad, sterile drapes, tampon, swabs, toothed forceps, scissors, needle holder)
- 20 ml syringe, needle; 20 ml 1% lignocaine, sharps box
- Warm tap water, lubricant
- Sterile gloves
- Waste bag

Salmon (1999) describes how women in her study used alarming words including 'torture' to describe their experience of suturing. In a descriptive study, Sanders et al (2002) reported that out of 68 women only 33% experienced no pain during suturing, and that 4.5% found it 'distressing', 7.5% 'horrible' and 4.5% 'excruciating'. A local anaesthetic will be required unless the woman has an epidural in situ. If the effects of the epidural have worn off, the woman should be consulted regarding the potential use of another top-up or local anaesthetic.

A total dose of up to 20 ml of 1% lignocaine can be infiltrated into the perineum (NICE 2007) (see Box 11.3). If the woman had a local anaesthetic prior to an episiotomy, then this amount should be included in the total amount

given. Inhalational analgesia can be a valuable source of relaxation during infiltration. Adequate analgesia is essential before this procedure is attempted, and the midwife or student attending must be the woman's advocate in this respect. Box 11.3 describes the procedure for administering local anaesthesia.

Which suture material?

In a systematic review of the evidence comparing synthetic suture material with catgut (Kettle & Johanson 1999), eight randomized trials were considered. The reviewers concluded that synthetic material gave rise to less pain in the first three postnatal days than catgut, resulting in the need for less analgesia. There was also less separation of the wound

Box 11.3 Infiltration of the perineum with local anaesthetic

Visualizing the perineal wound as a diamond shape, insert the needle at the left or right lateral point upwards towards the top point of the diamond (vaginal wall). Inject local anaesthetic as the needle is steadily withdrawn back to the point of initial insertion. Keeping the needle in position and reversing its direction, insert it along the perineal aspect of the wound, towards the bottom point of the diamond. Again, inject the lignocaine as the needle is withdrawn back towards the site of initial insertion. Remove the needle and repeat this process along the other side of the wound.

Before starting the suturing, the effectiveness of the anaesthesia should be checked, giving time for the local anaesthetic to take effect.

(dehiscence) in this group although there was no difference in the amount of dyspareunia experienced by women or reports of long-term perineal pain.

Standard synthetic material, however, takes longer to dissolve than catgut and is associated with the need for suture removal up to 3 months after the birth (Mahomed et al 1989). A synthetic suture material that dissolves more rapidly than standard material has now been developed. In a trial comparing the new material with the standard material for women following spontaneous vaginal birth (Kettle et al 2002), it was concluded that the rate of suture removal was significantly lower in women sutured with the new material, and there was no difference between groups regarding pain 10 days after the birth.

Assisting during perineal suturing

Students are often asked to assist the person suturing the perineum by adding equipment to the sterile field, enabling the procedure to progress without interruption. The student can open the sterile syringe onto the sterile field by peeling back the paper covering halfway and holding it over the trolley for the midwife or doctor to grasp. The needle and suture material can also be opened and dropped onto the sterile field. The lignocaine should be checked for correct concentration, expiry date and that the solution is clear before being inverted and held for the person suturing to access.

A light-hearted atmosphere should be maintained and the baby held close to its mother, preferably by the woman's birth partner. They can continue to share their exploration of the baby, as the procedure should not be painful once the initial infiltration is over. The student should observe the woman's face for any signs of discomfort, and ask her how she is feeling. Any pain or concern should be reported back to the practitioner undertaking the procedure.

Suture technique

Current evidence from a systematice
review (Kettle et al 2007) suggests that
the most appropriate technique for
repairing perineal damage following
childbirth is a continuous, non-locking
suture to align vaginal wall mucosa and
then perineal muscle. This technique
is favoured over the use of interrupted
sutures. Care should be taken to reduce
any dead space as this could allow
blood to leak into it, increasing the risk
of haematoma formation, pain and
infection. Where the skin is opposed,
this should not be sutured. If suturing
of the skin is required this should
be using a continuous, sub-cuticular
technique (NICE 2007). The use of
a continuous suturing technique is
associated with less pain for up to
10 days postpartum (Morano et al
2006) and a reduction in dyspareunia,
although a subsequent randomized
trial concluded that interrupted
sutures with inverted knots resulted
in similar outcomes to the continuous
suture method (Kindberg et al 2008).
Continuous suturing is however quicker
and this technique therefore reduces the
length of time the woman is exposed
during this intimate procedure.

Analgesia following perineal repair

The perineum can be a significant
source of pain in the postnatal period,
making it difficult for the woman to
undertake important activities, for

Activity

Practise using a needle holder by
taping half a sanitary towel to the back
of a chair and suturing this makeshift
'perineum'.

Practise knots by tying a length of
string around your leg, just above the
knee.

example, breastfeeding (Montgomery
2000). In a systematic review assessing
the effectiveness of non-steroidal anti-
inflammatory drugs (NSAIDs) given
rectally following perineal trauma after
childbirth (Hedayati et al 2004), three
trials were considered. The reviewers
concluded that NSAID suppositories
resulted in less pain in the first 24 hours
following the birth and reduced the
need for additional analgesia during that
time. NICE intrapartum care guidelines
therefore recommend the use of a rectal
non-steroidal anti-inflammatory drug
following perineal repair of first- and
second-degree trauma (NICE 2007:39).
Cool maternity gel pads can provide
local relief (Steen et al 2000).

Activity

Find out which drugs are offered
to women where you work to help
alleviate perineal pain after birth.

What suture material have you seen
used for perineal repair?

Find out about the content of the
training programme for midwives
to gain or maintain competence in
perineal repair where you work.

Reflection on trigger

Look back on the trigger scenario.

Penny held her baby close and kissed her forehead, breathing in her smell and warmth. Her baby was finally here. The hard work of the last countless hours had come to an end. She looked up at her husband, who was cradling them both. They exchanged smiles and explored their daughter's tiny fingers and fine dark hair. They talked to her gently. 'I'm afraid you're going to need stitches,' the midwife said.

Now that you are familiar with the procedure for perineal suturing you should have insight into how the scenario relates to the evidence about this procedure. The jigsaw model will now be used to explore the trigger scenario in more depth.

Effective communication

It is important that the midwife explains to the woman why she feels that suturing is indicated and the extent of the damage, taking into account who else is listening to this information when she describes the detail. The midwife can use this opportunity to reassure the woman that the perineum has a fantastic blood supply which enables it to heal quickly. She should also reassure the woman that she will ensure that the area is anaesthetized before she begins to suture. Questions that arise from the scenario might include: What information had Penny received antenatally about trauma to the perineum? How might

the need for suturing have been phrased differently? What written information is available where you work regarding care of a sutured perineum in the postnatal period?

Woman-centred care

The woman is key to the planning of care. She should be involved at all stages and understand the rationale behind the care she receives. The plan should be regularly reviewed and discussed with her in the light of her current health status. Questions that arise from the scenario might include: Has Penny documented anything in her birth plan about perineal care? How can she be involved in decisions about her perineal care? What factors need to be considered to ensure that any advice offered to Penny meets her individual needs? Have her wishes for contact with her baby been upheld or disrupted in any way because of the need for suturing?

Using best evidence

Midwives have a duty to provide care based on the best available evidence (NMC 2008). The evidence should therefore be reviewed systematically and discussed with the multi-professional team, leading to the development of appropriate local clinical guidelines. Questions that arise from the scenario might include: What is the most appropriate suturing technique to ensure that the perineum heals with least impact on subsequent pain during sexual intercourse? What does the evidence say about antenatal perineal massage for reducing perineal trauma? Is this reflected in the local policy? What evidence supports the use of sub-cuticular suturing to the skin layer? What is the most appropriate form of analgesia following perineal suturing?

Professional and legal issues

Perineal care is part of the midwife's role and has the potential to impact on the woman's health and wellbeing for years to come. It is essential that the midwife acknowledges her accountability and seeks informed consent for all treatment and care involved in this intimate aspect of her practice. Questions that arise from the scenario might include: What should the midwife do if she feels that the perineal repair is beyond her clinical competence? What action should the midwife take if Penny refuses suturing? How can the midwife maintain her skills in perineal suturing? What are the key components of comprehensive documentation of the procedure?

Team working

The midwife must acknowledge the limits of her professional competence and seek support from senior members of the team if she feels that the repair is beyond her expertise. She should also engage the expertise of other professionals if the woman could potentially benefit from additional care, for example, perineal ultrasound. Questions that arise from the scenario might include: Which other members

of the healthcare team have skills that might enhance the woman's recovery from perineal trauma? What is the process for referral to another healthcare professional where you work? Is the midwife accountable for the care given by another healthcare professional?

Clinical dexterity

Repair of the perineum requires considerable dexterity. It is a skill that is initiated during pre-registration education and consolidated throughout professional clinical practice. Questions that arise from the scenario might include: What opportunities were available for the midwife to learn how to suture the perineum when she was a student midwife? How did she develop her skills in perineal suturing? How was her competence verified and maintained? Is there a mechanism for the midwife to audit the effectiveness of her perineal suturing skills? Will the midwife consider suturing without the use of stirrups and lithotomy position?

Models of care

The way that postpartum perineal care is provided may vary depending on the models of care practised. For example, where there is a low prevalence of home births, community midwives may not have had the opportunity to develop or maintain their suturing skills. Questions that arise from the scenario might include: How does the place of birth impact on the availability of perineal suturing by the midwife who was present at the birth? If the birth took place in a midwifery-led unit, how would the midwife access senior advice if required? What are the advantages and disadvantages of giving birth in a hospital for women who require perineal suturing?

Safe environment

Ensuring that women feel that their privacy and dignity are maintained is an essential part of helping them feel safe and secure. Women are particularly exposed during perineal suturing and it is important to provide them with reassurance that they will not be disturbed during the procedure. Questions that arise from the scenario might include: How will the midwife ensure that no-one else enters the room during the suturing process? What is the role of the birth partner during perineal suturing? When should consent be gained for the post-procedure administration of an anti-inflammatory suppository? How will the midwife ensure that no swabs or needles are unaccounted for at the end of the procedure?

Promotes health

Throughout the provision of midwifery care there are many opportunities to promote maternal health. It is a time when women can be given information that enables them to make decisions and take actions that can enhance both their physical and emotional wellbeing. Questions that arise from the scenario might include: What information can the midwife provide to facilitate

perineal healing? How can such information be reinforced and made meaningful for Penny? What advice should Penny be given about resuming sexual intercourse following the birth and when is the most appropriate time to offer such advice?

Further scenarios

The following scenarios enable you to consider how specific situations influence the care the midwife provides. Use the jigsaw model to explore the issues raised in each scenario.

Scenario 1

Fatima is a 20-year-old woman who had infibulation when she was 12 years old. Prior to the birth it was necessary to surgically de-infibulate to allow the unobstructed birth of her baby. After the birth her husband requests that she is 'closed up' again.

Practice point

Female genital mutilation (FGM) is widely practised in many African, middle and south-east Asian countries. However, it is outlawed in this country under the Female Genital Mutilation (England, Wales and Northern Ireland) Act 2003.

Further questions specific to Scenario 1 include:

1. Is the midwife obliged to agree to his request?
2. Who should she access for support with this issue?

3. What mechanisms can help midwives explore controversial issues?

4. What are the potential consequences for the woman if the request is turned down?

5. Is there a midwife where you work who has a special interest in FGM?

6. What are the health risks associated with this procedure?

7. What are the child protection issues this practice raises?

Scenario 2

You are observing your mentor prepare to suture the woman that you have just supported throughout her birth. Following examination after the delivery of the placenta, you identified that she had sustained a second-degree tear. The woman had an epidural during the first stage of labour but this has now worn off. The midwife starts to suture and the woman shouts 'Ouch, I can feel that.'

Practice point

It is important that the woman is pain-free when the perineum is being sutured so that she can relax. This enables her to keep still and for the wound to be accurately viewed and repaired. It is also important that she is free from pain as this is a very sensitive area of her anatomy and to inflict pain would be an abuse of her.

Further questions specific to Scenario 2 include:

1. What should the student midwife do?

2. What options are available for pain relief during perineal suturing?

3. How long do the different methods take to work?

4. How can the student help the woman relax during suturing?

5. What is the most appropriate time for women to have their perineum sutured after the birth?

6. When might suturing need to be delayed or expediated?

Conclusion

Student midwives must make the most of their pre-registration opportunity to observe many skilled practitioners undertake this important repair. They also have the potential to make a positive difference to women's experience of perineal suturing by being their advocate and companion during this intimate procedure.

The skill and techniques employed by the midwife or doctor who assesses and cares for the woman following perineal trauma can have a significant impact on her recovery. The most appropriate method of repair is a continuous, non-locking suture to the vaginal wall, followed by repair of the perineal muscles. If the skin edges do not then lie close together, they should be brought together with a sub-cuticular stitch. If a midwife feels that a perineal wound is beyond her expertise, she should refer to a senior obstetrician rather than to a house officer. All complicated tears should be referred to a senior practitioner.

Resources

Association of Radical Midwives. The perineum and perineal tears: http://www.radmid.demon.co.uk/perineum.htm.

Beckmann M, Garrett A: Antenatal perineal massage for reducing perineal trauma, *Cochrane Database of Systematic Reviews* 2006, (CD005123).

Johnson R, Taylor W: *Skills for midwifery practice*, ed 2, Edinburgh, 2006, Elsevier. Ch. 37, pp. 283-298.

Wickham S: With woman – perineal pampering: http://www.withwoman.co.uk/contents/info/perineal.html. July 1, 2008.

Women's Health Specialist Library: Royal College of Midwives evidence-based guidelines. Suturing the perineum: http://www.library.nhs.uk/womenshealth/ViewResource.aspx?resID = 82619.

References

Dahlen H, Homer C: What are the views of midwives in relation to perineal repair? *Women and Birth: Journal of the Australian College of Midwives* 21(1): 27–35, 2008.

Female Genital Mutilation Act: Ch. 31, 2003. Online. Available http://www.opsi.gov.uk/ACTS/acts2003/ukpga_20030031_en_1. December 11, 2008.

Fleming EM, Hagen S, Niven C: Does perineal suturing make a difference? The SUNS trial, *British Journal of Obstetrics and Gynaecology* 110(7):684–689, 2003.

Gordon B, Mackrodt C, Fern E, et al: The Ipswich Childbirth Study: a randomised evaluation of two stage postpartum perineal repair leaving the skin unsutured, *British Journal of Obstetrics and Gynaecology* 105: 435–440, 1998.

Grant A, Gordon B, Mackrodat C, et al: The Ipswich childbirth study: one year follow up of alternative methods used in perineal repair, *British Journal of Obstetrics and Gynaecology* 108(1): 34–40, 2001.

Hedayati H, Parsons J, Crowther CA: Rectal analgesia for pain from perineal trauma following childbirth (Cochrane Review). In *The Cochrane Library, Issue 1*, Chichester, 2004, John Wiley.

Kettle C, Johanson RB: Absorbable synthetic versus catgut suture material for perineal repair. DOI: 10.1002/14651858.CD000006, *Cochrane Database of Systematic Reviews* 3, 1999 (CD000006).

Kettle C, Hills RK, Jones P, et al: Continuous versus interrupted perineal repair with standard or rapidly absorbed sutures after spontaneous vaginal birth: a randomised controlled trial, *The Lancet* 359:2217–2223, 2002.

Kettle C, Hills RK, Ismail KMK: Continuous versus interrupted sutures for repair of episiotomy or second degree tears. DOI: 10.1002/14651858. CD000947.pub2, *Cochrane Database of Systematic Reviews* 3, 2007 (CD000947).

Kindberg S, Stehouwer M, Hvidman L, et al: Postpartum perineal repair performed by midwives: a randomised trial comparing two suture techniques leaving the skin unsutured, *BJOG: an International Journal of Obstetrics & Gynaecology* 115(4): 472–479, 2008.

Mahomed K, Grant A, Ashurst HM, et al: The Southmead perineal suture study: a randomised comparison of suture materials and suturing techniques for repair of perineal trauma, *British Journal of Obstetrics and Gynaecology* 96:1272–1280, 1989.

Montgomery A: Breastfeeding and postpartum maternal care, *Primary Care* 27(1):237–250, 2000.

Morano S, Mistrangelo E, Pastorino D, et al: A randomized comparison of suturing techniques for episiotomy and laceration repair after spontaneous vaginal birth, *Journal of Minimal Invasive Gynecology* 13(5):457–462, 2006.

National Institute for Health and Clinical Excellence (NICE): *Intrapartum care. Care of healthy women and their babies during childbirth. NICE clinical guideline 55*, London, 2007, NICE.

Nursing and Midwifery Council (NMC): *Midwives rules and standards*, London, 2004, NMC.

Nursing and Midwifery Council (NMC): *The Code. Standards of conduct, performance and ethics for nurses and midwives*, London, 2008, NMC.

Nursing and Midwifery Council (NMC): *Standards for pre-registration midwifery education*, London, 2009, NMC.

Oboro VO, Tabowei TO, Loto OM, et al: A multicentre evaluation of the two layer repair of postpartum perineal trauma, *Journal of Obstetrics and Gynaecology* 1:5–8, 2003.

Salmon D: A feminist analysis of women's experiences of perineal trauma in the immediate post-delivery period, *Midwifery* 15:247–256, 1999.

Sanders J, Campbell R, Peters TJ: Effectiveness of pain relief during perineal suturing, *British Journal of Obstetrics and Gynaecology* 109: 1066–1068, 2002.

Steen M, Cooper K: A randomised controlled trial to compare the effectiveness of icepacks and Epifoam with cooling maternity gel pads at alleviating postnatal perineal trauma, *Midwifery* 16(1):48–55, 2000.

Index